MW01230521

CLUSTER HEADACHE

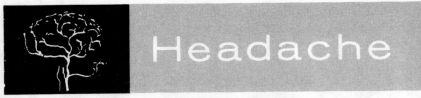

OFFICIAL PUBLICATION OF THE AMERICAN
ASSOCIATION FOR THE STUDY OF HEADACHE

CLUSTER HEADACHE

EDITED BY

NINAN T. MATHEW, M.D.

DIRECTOR, HOUSTON HEADACHE CLINIC

AND

DEPARTMENT OF NEUROLOGY

UNIVERSITY OF TEXAS

MEDICAL SCHOOL

HOUSTON, TEXAS

SP

SP MEDICAL & SCIENTIFIC BOOKS
a division of Spectrum Publications, Inc.
New York

SPECTRUM PUBLICATIONS, INC.
175-20 Wexford Terrace
Jamaica, NY 11432

Library of Congress Cataloging in Publication Data
Main entry under title:

Cluster headache.

    Bibliography: p.
    Includes index.
    1. Cluster headache. I. Mathew, Ninan T. [DNLM:
1. Vascular headache. WL 344 C649]
RC392.C58 1984   616.8'4   84-4925
ISBN 0-89335-204-7

Printed in the United States of America

Contributors

J. Keith Campbell, MD • Department of Neurology, Mayo Clinic, Rochester, Minnesota

James R. Couch, Jr., MD • Chief, Division of Neurology, Southern Illinois University School of Medicine, Springfield, Illinois

Donald J. Dalessio, MD • Chairman, Department of Medicine, Scripps Clinical Medical Group, Inc., La Jolla, California

James D. Dexter, MD • Chairman, Department of Neurology, University of Missouri School of Medicine, Columbia, Missouri

Seymour Diamond, MD • Department of Pharmacology, Chicago Medical School; Director, Diamond Headache Clinic, Chicago, Illinois

John Edmeads, MD • Chief of Neurology, Sunnybrook Medical Center; President, American Association for the Study of Headache, Toronto, Ontario

Arnold P. Friedman, MD • Department of Neurology, University of Arizona School of Medicine, Tuscon, Arizona

John R. Graham, MD • Director, Headache Research Foundation, Faulkner Hospital, Boston, Massachusetts

Robert S. Kunkel, MD • The Cleveland Clinic Foundation, Cleveland, Ohio

Ninan T. Mathew, MD • Director, Houston Headache Clinic; Department of Neurology, University of Texas Medical School, Houston, Texas

Joel R. Saper, MD • Department of Neurology, Michigan State University Medical School; Director, Michigan Headache and Neurological Institute, Ann Arbor, Michigan

William G. Speed III, MD • Department of Medicine, Johns Hopkins University Medical School; Speed Headache Associates, Baltimore, Maryland

N. Vijayan, MD • Sacramento Headache and Neurology Clinic, Sacramento, California

Craig Watson, MD, PhD • Sacramento Headache and Neurology Clinic, Sacramento, California.

Foreword

This book constitutes a compilation and integration of the latest advances in the management of cluster headaches. It encompasses the work of nine experts in the field of headache in the U.S. and presents a thorough and comprehensive view of the subject. Most of the participants at the symposium have spent years studying cluster headache and its variants. They present a variety of conceptions in a comprehensive manner. It is believed that the generalist, neurologist, or other medical specialist involved in the treatment of this difficult syndrome will derive diagnostic and therapeutic insight into its management. The patients seeking help and understanding of their condition will be the ultimate beneficiaries of its information.

SEYMOUR DIAMOND, M.D.
March, 1984

Preface

The past decade has witnessed a surge of interest in the field of headache and related disorders. Even though the pathophysiology and pathogenesis of primary headache disorders are still poorly understood, recent clinical and therapeutic observations have greatly contributed to improvement of patient care in the headache field. Headache clinics specializing in the diagnosis and comprehensive management of headaches, now available in most major cities, have also helped in the progress of patient care and research.

Cluster headache, being one of the most severe forms of headache and probably the most "pure" form of headache, deserves special attention. The American Association for the Study of Headache has planned a series of advanced courses in certain aspects of headache and chose cluster headache as the first topic to be discussed. In this advanced course, the faculty was selected because of their special experience in treating cluster headaches and their wider experience in the field of headache research and therapy. This monograph is an outgrowth of that course. Historical aspects of cluster headache are very adequately dealt with by Dr. William Speed. John Graham has painstakingly compared migraine and cluster headache and brought out their differences and similarities. The section on therapy is dealt with by physicians who have first-hand experience in treating a large number of patients with cluster headache, and who are also researchers in that particular aspect of the disease. The controversial treatments like histamine desensitization is dealt with by a respected member of the Neurology Department of the Mayo Clinic, where this form of treatment originated years ago.

Overall, this book gives a balanced view of a number of specialists in the field rather than a fixed view of one individual author, and is the first of a series on various aspects of headache.

Ninan T. Mathew, M.D.

Contents

Contributors   v

Foreword   vii

Preface   ix

Chapter 1
History, Nomenclature, Relation to Other Facial
Pain Syndromes   1
William G. Speed III

Chapter 2
Classification of Cluster Headache: Clinical Features
of Episodic Cluster Headache   15
Robert S. Kunkel

Chapter 3
Variants of Cluster Headache   21
Seymour Diamond

Chapter 4
Nonheadache Disorders and Characteristics of Cluster
Headache Patients   31
Joel R. Saper

Chapter 5
Peripheral Autonomic Abnormalities in Cluster Headache   45
N. Vijayan and Craig Watson

Chapter 6
Pathyphysiologic Aspects of Cluster Headache   57
John Edmeads

Chapter 7
Cycles in Cluster Headache   69
James D. Dexter

Chapter 8
The Psychological and Behavioral Aspects of the
Cluster Headache Patient   73
Arnold P. Friedman

Chapter 9
The Relation of Cluster Headache to Migraine   79
John R. Graham

Chapter 10
Treatment and Management of Acute Cluster Headache   89
James R. Couch, Jr.

Chapter 11
Prophylactic Pharmacotherapy of Cluster Headache   97
Ninan T. Mathew

Chaper 12
The Current Status of Histamine Desensitization in the
Treatment of Cluster Headache   111
J. Keith Campbell

Chapter 13
Surgical Therapy of Cluster Headache   119
Donald J. Dalessio

Chapter 14
Cluster Headache: The Treatment-Resistant Patient   127
J. Keith Campbell

Index   135

CLUSTER HEADACHE

1
History, Nomenclature, Relation to Other Facial Pain Syndromes

WILLIAM G. SPEED III

Claims for the first description of cluster headaches have been in dispute for years and we may never be certain who deserves the credit. Before one reviews the literature in search of the historical background of cluster headaches, it is necessary to establish acceptable clinical criteria. I have undertaken to do this by relying on my own personal experience with cluster headache and on many of the criteria published in the literature.[1-9]

These criteria are:

1. Unilateral head pain around, in or behind the eye, temple, forehead, which may include the maxilla, and may spread to the mandible, upper and/or lower teeth, and possibly the neck. Extension of the pain more posteriorly in the head would not exclude the diagnosis, but unilateral posterior headache without the anterior portion should not be considered a manifestation of cluster headache.

2. Frequency: one to four attacks per 24 hours.

3. Duration: 10–240 minutes.

4. The headache may be accompanied by nasal congestion, rhinorrhea, lacrimation, and conjunctival injection.

5. The headache may be accompanied by homolateral miosis and ptosis of the upper lid.

6. Attacks may be diurnal and/or nocturnal.

7. Character of the pains: throbbing, pounding, boring, pressing, burning, sharp or stabbing.

8. Cycles, clusters, or groups of these headaches, lasting for weeks or months followed by similar periods of remissions, are characteristic of episodic cluster headache as we know it today, but the absence of these clusters in the historical review of the literature was not considered critical since the cluster phenomenon can be recognized by the characteristics of the individual attacks of headache.

Admittedly, we have seen variations from the above criteria but I believe that these represent the nucleus of what we consider the clinical picture of cluster headaches to be. If that is the case, then certain conclusions concerning the first description can be drawn from a review of the medical literature.

Some authors[10,11] have attributed the first description to Benjamin Hutchinson of Great Britain who in 1822 reported on cases of neuralgia spasmodica.[11,12] He reported on 28 cases, none of which meet the above criteria. However, on page 28 of this document, Hutchinson makes the following comment: "Hartenkeil, Hildebrande, Baldinger, and some other German writers, relate cases of what they call Tic Douloureux; which, though in some particulars they resemble that affection, in others differ from it very materially. The first of these writers describes it as having been very prevalent at Salzburg: but the pain was periodical, recurring once in 24 hours; often remaining for several hours at a time, and then suddenly departing." This sketchy comment might refer to a description of cluster headache but it is really inadequate to accept this as the first description; Hutchinson himself attributed such a report to others. Unfortunately, he did not give references and the original source to which he referred could not be found. A review of Hutchinson's other case presentation in this treatise indicates that they are essentially those of Tic Douloureux and not cluster headache. Therefore, with all due respect to our British colleagues, it is not established that Benjamin Hutchinson presented the first description.

Some authors[2,4,11,13] give credit to Moritz Heinric Romberg, Professor of Medicine at the University of Berlin. In his book written in 1840, entitled *A Manual of the Nervous Diseases of Man,*[14] under the heading Ciliary Neuralgia, he states the following: "Painful sensations in the eye, which are generally confined to one side, and are excited or incrreased by rays of light and by visual efforts, are the characteristic symptoms of this affection. In the higher degrees photophobia is present; this is therefore the term generally applied to the affection. The patient avoids solar and artificial light, as the bulb of the eye becomes painful when exposed to their influence, and the eyelids contract painfully. The pupil is contracted. The pain not unfrequently extends over the head and face. The eye generally weeps and becomes red. These symptoms occur in paroxysms, of a uniform or irregular character, and isolated or combined with facial neuralgia and hemicrania." Is that a description of cluster headache? I suppose it could be, but it differs in one striking way from what we see in cluster headache today and that is Dr. Romberg's comment regarding the high degree of photophobia in the condition he described. This I believe is unusual in cluster headache. I found "ciliary neuralgia," as Romberg described it, the most difficult one to decide as to whether or not he was describing cluster headache. Perhaps, but there are reservations. In 1867, Möllendorff published[15] an account of a new syndrome which some have felt was an early description of cluster headache.[8,16,17] However, a careful review of his comments indicate that he is describing migraine. He found the attacks occuring mostly in women at the time of menses, and that the attacks had some relation to emotional disturbances. The attacks began with a light in the eye and rotating spots and he described the pain as shifting from one side to the other and noted it was better when lying flat. These are not features of cluster headache.

In 1878, Albert Eulenburg, Professor of Neurology at the University of Greifswold, in his textbook *Lehrbuch der Dervenkrankheiten* described headaches which he called hemicrania angioparalytica or neuroparalytica.[18] He stated that in this form, at the peak of the attack, the painful side is reddish, hot, and the conjunctiva is injected; there is an increased production of tears and the pupil is contracted. Occasionally there is a narrowing of the lid, retraction of the bulb, and the upper lid is drooping. The ear is reddish and hot and the production of sweat is increased; the temporal artery is dilated and the carotid artery pulsations on the painful side are stronger. The pulse rate is slowed to 48–56 per minute. The duration of the paroxysmal attacks varies from a few hours to a half a day, rarely lasting for a whole day or several days, with alternating remissions and exacerbations. With slow dimunution of the pain, the patient feels exhausted, falls asleep and may awaken feeling well. Was Eulenburg describing cluster headache? H. Heych[19] argues strongly that he was because he gave a description of hemicrania with tear formation, Horner's Syndrome: warming of the skin, hyperhidrosis, bradycardia and the vascular origin of the pain. I agree with Heych's comment but Eulenburg clearly states that the attacks vary from a few hours to half a day and rarely to an entire day or several days. The duration of a half a day, entire day, or several days is unlike that of cluster headache. However in fairness to Eulenburg, since he did state that the long durations were rare, he should be given a "probable" as the first describer of cluster headache. It certainly is the closest description one finds in the 19th century literature.

In 1910 and 1912, Greenfield Sluder of Washington University, St Louis, Missouri[20] described a syndrome that has been confused with cluster headache. He described sphenopalatine ganglion neuralgia as a pain at the root of the nose and in and about the eye and upper jaw and teeth extending backward under the zygoma to the ear and to the mastoid with the severest pain often at a point five centimeters back of the mastoid extending then to the neck, shoulder blade, breast and when severe, to the arm, forearm, hand and fingers, and sometimes a sense of sore throat on that side. In some he described a motor phenomenon such as an arching of the soft palette on the affected side and the uvula inclined obliquely to the well side. I believe Sluder can be excluded as a describer of cluster headache.

In 1912, R. Bing[21] coined the term erythroprosopalgia (erythro (red) + prosopon (face) + algia (pain), a nervous disorder analagous to erythromelalgia (erythro (red) + melos (limb) + algia (Pain)). The latter is a disease affecting chiefly the extremities (feet more often than hands) and it is marked by paroxysmal bilateral vasodilatation with burning pain in the face and causing severe recurring headaches. Bing's description emphasized autonomic features rather then pain. This is probably not a description of cluster headache.

In 1925, Vallery-Radot and Blamontier[22,23] of France wrote about a 38-year old female with recurrent severe unilateral right sided headache and homolateral lacrimation and rhinorrhea. Unfortunately, they did not comment on the frequency or duration patterns of these headaches or the location of the pains. They did recognize the vascular nature of the headache they were describing by calling it the "syndrome de vasodilatation hemicephalique d'origine sympathique". The authors may well have described cluster headache but because their data lacks significant detail one can consider this only a possible description.

In 1926, Wilfred Harris[24] of Great Britain devoted a section of his book, *Neuritis and Neuralgia*, to the description of a condition to which he gave the name, "periodic migrainous neuralgia". He described a syndrome consisting of recurrent attacks of excruciating, severe, unilateral, knife-like pain extending from the outer canthus of the eye and from the hairline, passing into the forehead at the side of the face, head and neck. The pain lasted from ten minutes to several hours recurring with remarkable regularity several times within 24 hours, including attacks which woke the patient about 3 AM. During the attack there was reddening and running of the affected eye. This sequence of events would be repeated every day for several weeks and the symptoms would then disappear for months, only to recur at a similar season the following year. This description clearly fits our concept of cluster headache today. Although others before Harris may have been describing the same syndrome, these descriptions were sufficiently imprecise (except possibly for Eulenburg) to leave a seed of doubt. Harris[25] confused the issue in an article in the British Medical Journal in 1936 in which he used the term "ciliary neuralgia", to describe a mixture of headaches; some of which were cluster, some migraine and some atypical facial neuralgia.

In 1931, Walter Dandy[26] of Johns Hopkins reported on the treatment of hemicrania by removal of the inferior cervical and first thoracic sympathetic ganglion. The first case of the two he presented was a 50-year-old man with recurrent bouts of headaches since the age of 17 involving right frontal, orbital and maxillary regions occurring once or as much as six times a day and lasting for a half an hour. The patient experienced unilateral ptosis, sweating, congestion of the conjunctiva, swelling of the nasal mucous membrane, fullness of the vessels of the face and bradycardia (pp. 40-50). Although Dandy felt these were migraine, the attacks he described are compatible with cluster headache. He appears therefore to be the first U.S. physician to describe cluster headaches.

In 1932, Harris Vail[27] reported in the *Annals of Otology, Rhinology, and Laryngology,* a description of head and facial pain under the title, "Vidian neuralgia." He made the following statement: "comparing the symptoms of the cases which I report here with the case reported by Sluder, it would be seen that they are identical." He was not suggesting that he was reporting something different, but only that the Vidian nerve was responsible rather than the sphenopalatine ganglion. It was felt that Sluder's cases did not represent cluster headache; therefore, Vail's did not.

In 1939, Horton, MacLean and Craig[28] reported 84 cases of unilateral headache which they described as erythromelalgia of the head and which later was described by Horton[29] as histaminic cephalgia, and later by others as Horton's headache or Horton's syndrome.[30] Their article in 1939 represented the most clearcut, accurate and precise description of cluster headache presented thus far in the U.S. literature. It is of interest that they made no mention of the descrip-

given by Wilfred Harris thirteen years before under the name of periodic migrainous neuralgia. The Horton et al description was one of pain limited to one side of the head, described as constant, excruciating, burning and boring; it involved the eye, temple, neck and often the face. The duration of the headache occurred with clock-like regularity, particularly at night, the patient awakening with pain night after night and week after week at a certain hour. Although they found night pain to be characteristic, it was stated that pain during the waking hours was common. Remissions and exacerbations in many cases occurred spontaneously. They described injection of the conjunctiva, plugging of the nose, profuse watering of the eye and nose and flushing of the side of the face. They were the first to point out the relationship of alcoholic beverages to exacerbations of pain in some cases.

In 1964, Gardner, Stowell and Dullinger[31] from the Department of Neurosurgery at Cleveland Clinic, reported on three cases with the characteristics of cluster headache and they felt that these symptoms could be explained by periodic discharges of parasympathetic impulses over the greater superficial petrosal branch of the seventh nerve. They suggested that this syndrome be called "greater superficial petrosal neuralgia," but this term never had popular acceptance.

In 1954, Kunkle, Pfeiffer, Wilholt, and Hamrick[32] reported in the *North Carolina Medical Journal* on, "Recurrent Brief Headache in 'Cluster' Pattern." They reported thirty cases and although they may not be the first to recognize the cyclic nature of this disorder, it appears they were the first to use the term cluster headache. In 1958, Friedman and Mikropoulos[8] from the Headache Unit of the Montefiore Hospital in New York City published in Neurology an article titled "Cluster Headaches." Following this, the term cluster headache became generally accepted and was recognized by the AD HOC Committee on Classification of Headache[33] from the National Institute of Neurological Diseases and Blindness in 1962, and by the World Federation of Neurology at the meeting of the research group on migraine and headache in 1969.[34]

In 1956, Sir Charles Symonds,[35] in *Brain* reported a series of 17 cases which had the characteristics of cluster headache. These were described under the term "a particular variety of headache."

Although Symonds states that many of the features of the headaches described in his communication are accurately portrayed in Horton's papers and the papers of Kunkle, Pfeiffer, Wilholt and Hamrick, it is his opinion that the diagnostic boundaries of migraine and its variants are not clearly defined and there is little justification for the segregation of "cluster" headache as a distinct and isolated entity.

It would appear, however, that there are distinct differences between cluster headache and migraine and, until the etiology of each is more clearly established, it would seem that the term cluster headache would be the most appropriate to use. It has been preferred in the literature for the past twenty eight years and I think the time has come to call a halt to other descriptive terms for this condition, at least until a specific etiology becomes established. This descriptive term obviously is not ideal. We know clearly that not all cluster headaches cluster.[36,37] Even though it appears that the British, through Harris, have the strongest claim to the first clear description of this disorder, I hope for the sake of ending a prolonged confusion of terms that we can agree to continue to use the term "cluster headache."

RELATIONSHIP OF OTHER CEPHALIC PAIN SYNDROMES TO CLUSTER HEADACHE:

Raeder's Paratrigeminal Syndrome

In 1924, Raeder[38] published a paper in which he described a syndrome of unilateral head pain including drooping of the eyelid and contracted pupil, ie, signs of oculosympathetic nerve involvement without loss of sweating of the face. He pointed out that the lesion must be at the base of the middle fossa and involves the oculosympathetic fibers which lie in the wall of the internal carotid artery and first division of fifth nerve. He called this the paratrigeminal syndrome. It was thought to have no etiological significance and was of value merely in localizing the process.

In 1958, F. R. Ford and F. D. Walsh[39] reported 25 cases in which only pain above the eye and occulosympathetic phenomenon were present. Males were affected more frequently than females. The first symptom was severe, throbbing pain located above one eye or the other. The pain usually occurred in the morning and frequently ceased about noon. It persisted for a number of weeks or even several months. They stressed that this was not Horner's syndrome as there was no loss of sweating of the face. After months, possibly a year, the lid lifts and the pupil expands to its normal size. They reported a few cases in which a second attack occurred. Although Raeder regarded it merely as an anatomical syndrome implicating a process at the base of the middle fossa, Ford and Walsh were impressed with the stereotyped character of the syndrome and suspected that it was usually due to a specific cause. They had not encountered an aneurysm, intracranial neoplasm, or subarachnoid hemorrhage. When their patients were carefully questioned, a clear history of throbbing morning headaches of many years duration, often associated with nausea and vomiting, was found. Unfortunately, they reported on only one case out of the more than 25 cases that they observed, stating that it seemed unnecessary to publish a series of case histories as they were all alike. However, the one they selected to report apparently differed because there were two attacks. One attack on the left side and another attack on the right side. Their description is too sketchy to be certain of the diagnosis but it is most suggestive of migraine. In the same year, in the *American Journal of Ophthalmology*, J. Lawton Smith[40] reported a series of eight cases considered to be Raeder's partrigeminal neuralgia. An analysis of these cases shows that they were compatible with cluster headache and one appeared to be migraine. The other three could not be classified from the data given, although two of them were associated with hypertension. Boniuk and Schlezinger[41] in 1961 published nine cases of Raeder's partrigeminal syndrome in which they postulated the concept that some of these cases resulted from an infectious process of obscure origin with localized intracranial involvement of the carotid sympathetic plexus. They suggest that in order to clarify the pathogenesis, prognosis and treatment of this syndrome it would be desirable to separate it into two groups.

Group I would include those cases with parasellar cranial nerve involvement such as those described in Raeder's original article. Group II would inlcude those without parasellar cranial nerve involvement. All of the reported cases in the English literature fall into this latter group. The disorder in the latter group appears to be relatively benign rather than a potential surgical problem when compared with those having parasellar cranial nerve involvement.

It appears that the syndrome of unilateral head pain, ptosis and miosis without alteration in sweating, localizes a lesion to the anterior portion of the middle fossa. Most of these cases are due to vascular headache, either cluster or migraine, and in such instances it would be more appropriate to describe them in these terms. At best, the term Raeder's syndrome is confusing and it is probably best to avoid it except in those cases with the triad of unilateral frontal head pain, myosis and ptosis without evidence of cranial nerve involvement and in which diagnosis of migraine or cluster headaches cannot be made.

Chronic Paroxysmal Hemicrania

In 1976 Dr. Ottar Sjaastad and Inge Dale[42,43] presented a paper entitled "A New (?) Clinical Headache Entity 'Chronic Paroxysmal Hemicrania.'" A preliminary report had been given in 1974. The pain is described as always unilateral, never changing sides, maximal in the temporal maxillary regions and around the eye or in the back of the head. During the attacks the patient prefers to sit or pace the floor and the pain attacks are relatively short, around thirty minutes. They appear with almost clocklike regularity, usually at intervals of one to three hours, including awakening the patient at night and they are associated with recognized "modified cluster patterns" with more severe attacks for weeks and these may recur at intervals of weeks or months. Unilateral lacrimation, conjunctival injection, and nasal stenosis are present during the attacks. The characteristics of cluster headaches are present in these patients, but there are three rather distinct differences: (1) the patients are usually female, (2) the attacks are more frequent, generally more than eight per 24 hours, (3) there is a striking response to nonsteroidal, antiinflammatory medications. It seems appropriate to categorize this syndrome as a cluster variant.

Meniere's Syndrome and Cluster Headache

In 1965 Gordon J. Gilbert,[44] from the Veteran's Administration Hospital in West Haven, Connecticut, reported three cases which he felt represented Meniere's syndrome and cluster headaches occurring in a relationship that suggested, at least in some instances, that Meniere's syndrome represented a variation of cluster headache. He felt that these were the result of recurrent paroxysmal focal vasodilation producing vertigo in some and headaches in others. It was the clustering nature of the vertiginous attack similar to cluster headache that led to the suggestion that in some instances Meniere's may represent a cluster variant.

Cluster/Migraine

In 1977 Medina and Diamond[45] reported seven patients with vascular headache. Five of these had headaches with cluster characteristics but were preceded by neurologic manifestations commonly accepted as those of migraine (in these cases there were scotomata, unilateral weakness, unilateral paresthesia and photopsia). The other two patients had symptoms characteristic of migraine but occurred in cluster similar to cluster headache. It is therefore likely that a few examples occur in which there are manifestations of both cluster and migraine occurring simultaneously and in this paper may be classified as a cluster variant but they could also represent a migraine.

Atypical Facial Neuralgia

Another group of patients exhibit unilateral spread of pains from the nose, eye, cheek and ear, sometimes involving the neck. The attacks are recurrent and variable in duration and may be associated with swelling of the turbinates, rhinorrhea, nasal obstruction and mood changes. The pains are aching and seem to arise deep in the head, face or eye with considerable variation in the distribution of these pains. They do not seem to fit the categories more easily recognized in facial pain syndromes such as migraine and cluster headache. There may be multiple etiologies including pathology in the nose, eyes, teeth, sinuses and pharynx. For the most part, the mechanism is a vascular one and some undoubtedly are psychogenic. It is predominantly a diagnosis of exclusion made only after a careful history and physical examination. They are not likely to be confused with the distinct picture of cluster headache patients.

The typical facial neuralgias have short bursts of pain with definite trigger zones and should not be confused with the cluster syndrome.

Finally, the nomenclature for cluster headaches include two varieties:

1. Episodic: these are the common variety of cluster headaches which come and go in clusters, groups or cycles lasting for weeks or months with individual acute attacks of pain occuring generally one to three times a day, lasting for ten minutes to two to four hours.

2. Chronic cluster headache: these are a variety less common than the episodic one. These represent cluster headache with all of the manifestations of the episodic variety but there is an absence of significant periods of remission. Ekbom and Olivarius[37] considered cluster headaches to be of the chronic variety when there has been no remission for a year. However, since it is uncommon for episodic cluster headache to persist for more than three to four months, perhaps one might shorten this period to six months and consider those attacks longer than six months as representing chronic cluster headache. There are two subdivisions of this: (a) primary chronic cluster—referring to those patients who have never had episodic

cluster and (b) secondary chronic cluster—representing those patients whose chronic state was preceded by a history of episodic cluster headache.

In summary, the syndrome of cluster headache has been clearly recognized since 1926 when it was described by Harris and may have been described in the early 19th century. Case presentations of those reporting head and facial pain prior to Harris's description in 1926 are not supported by data sufficient to make it clear that they were describing cluster headache. Although Harris, in his description of "periodic migrainous neuralgia," clearly described cluster headache, those who have reported this syndrome since 1952 have consistently used the term cluster headache. For the sake of unity and an end to the confusion of terminology, it is suggested that we continue to use this term until a clear etiologic concept of this order is established.

Cluster headaches may occur as episodic, primary chronic, or secondary chronic. A few variants of this syndrome or closely related head and facial pains have been described.

REFERENCES

1. Dalessio, DJ: *Wolff's Headache and other Head Pain*, ed. 4. New York, Oxford University Press, 1980.
2. Kudrow L: *Cluster Headache and Mechanisms and Management.* New York, Oxford University Press, 1980.
3. Lance JW: *Headache Understanding Alleviation.* New York, Charles Scribner & Sons, 1975.
4. Lance JW: *Mechanism and Management of Headache*, ed 3. London-Boston, Butterworths, 1978.
5. Raskin NH, Appenzeller O: *Headache*, Vol XIX of *Major Problems in Internal Medicine.* Philadelphia, WB Saunders Co, 1980.
6. Diamond S, Dalessio DJ: *The Practicing Physician's Approach to Head-Ache*, ed 2. Baltimore, The Williams and Wilkins Co, 1978.
7. Robinson BW: Histaminic cephalgia. *Medicine*, 1958; 37:166-167.
8. Friedman, AP, Mikropoulos HE: Cluster headaches. *Neurology* 1958; 8:657-659.
9. Horton BT: Histaminic cephalgia: Differential diagnosis and treatment. *Proc Staff Meet Mayo Clin* 1956; 31:325–333.
10. Harrington E: *The Headache Book.* Connecticut, Technomatics Publications, 1980, p 25.
11. *Br. Med. J.* Editorial. 1975; 4:425-426.
12. Hutchinson B: *Cases of Neuralgia Spasmodicas Commonly Termed Tic Douloureux, Successfully Treated*, ed 4. London, Longman, 1822.
13. Diamond S: Cluster headache, relation to and comparison with migraine. *Postgrad Med* 1979; 66:87.

14. Romberg MH: *A Manual of Nervous Diseases of Man*, Sieveking (trans). 1:56 London, Syndenham Society, 1853.
15. Mollendorff: Ueber Hemikranie. *Vir Arch Path Anat* 1867; 41:385-395.
16. DuVoisin RE, Parker CW, Krenoyer WL: The cluster headache. *Arch Int Med* 1961; 108:111-116.
17. Eadie MJ, Sutherland JM: Migrainous Neuralgia. *Med J Aust* 1966; 53: 1053-1056.
18. Eulenburg A: Neuroses of sympathetic nerves. *Lehrbuch der Dervenkrankheiten* 1878; 2:264-274.
19. Heych H: Der cluster—kopfschmerz. *Deutsche Medizinische Wochenscheift* 1975; 100:1292-1293.
20. Sluder S: Etiology, diagnosis, prognosis and treatment of spenopaletine ganglion neuralgia. *JAMA* 1913; 61:1201-1205.
21. Bing R: *Lehrbuch der Nervenkrankheiten* Berlin, Urban and Schwarzenberg, 1913.
22. Vallery-Radot P, Blamontier P: Syndrome de Vasodilatation Hemicephalique d'origine Sympotique. *Bull Soc Med Hop* 1925; 49:1488-1493.
23. Vallery-Radot P, Wolfromm R, Barkizet J: Syndrome de Vaso-dilatation hemicephalique ou Cephalie Histaminique. *La Presse Medicole* 1951; 59: 499-500.
24. Harris W: Neuritis and Neuralgia. Oxford, Oxford University Press, 1926, pp 301-313.
25. Harris W: Ciliary (migrainous) neuralgia and its treatment. *Br Med J* 1936; 1:457-460.
26. Dandy WE: Treatment of hemicrania (migraine) by removal of the inferior cervical and first thoracic sympathetic ganglion. *Bull Johns Hop Hosp* 1931; 48:357-361.
27. Vail HH: Vidian neuralgia. *Ann Oto Rhin Laryngol*, 1932; 41:837-856.
28. Horton BT, MacLean AR, Craig WM: A new syndrome of vascular headache: Results of treatment with histamine: preliminary report. *Proc Staff Meet Mayo Clin* 14:257-260, 1939.
29. Horton BT: Histaminic cephalgia (Horton's Headache or Syndrome): provocative tests. *Triangle* 1957; 3:66-71.
30. Rapidis AD, et al: Horton's Syndrome. *Int J Oral Surg* 1977; 6:321-327.
31. Gardner WJ, Stowell A, Dullinger R: Resection of the greater superficial petrosal nerve in the treatment of unilateral headache. *J Neurosurg* 1947; 4:105.
32. Kunkle EC, Pfeiffer JB, Wilholt WM and Hamrick LD: Recurrent brief headache in "cluster" pattern. *Tr Am Neurol A* 1952; 77:240-243.
33. Ad Hoc Committee on classification of headache. *JAMA* 1962; 179:717-718.
34. World Federation of Neurology: *J Neurol Sci* 1969; 9:202.
35. Symonds C: A particular variety of headache. *Brain.* 1956; 79:217-232.
36. Rooke ED, Rushton JG, and Peters GA: Vasocilating headache: A suggestive classification and results of prophylactic treatment with UML 491 (methysergide). *Proc Staff Meet Mayo Clin* 1962; 37:433.
37. Ekbom K, Olivarius B: Chronic migrainous neuralgia—diagnostic and therapeutic aspects. *Headache* 1971; 11:97-101.
38. Raeder JG: Paratrigeminal paralysis of the oculopupillary sympathetic. *Brain* 1924; 47:149.

39. Ford FR, Walsh FB: Reader's paratrigeminal syndrome—a benign disorder, possibly a complication of migraine. *Bull J Hop H* 1958; 103:296-298.
40. Smith JL: Reader's partrigeminal syndrome. *Am J Ophth* 1958; 46:194-201.
41. Boniuk M, Schlezinger NS: Reader's paratrigeminal syndrome. *Am J Ophthal* 1962; 54:1074.
42. Sjaastad O, Dale I: Evidence for a new (?) treatable headache entity: A preliminary report. *Headache* 1974; 14:105-108.
43. Sjaastad O, Dale I: A new (?) clinical headache entity "Chronic Paroxysmal Hemicrania". *Acta Neurol Scand* 1976; 54:140-159.
44. Gilbert GJ: Meniere's syndrome and cluster headaches—recurrent paroxysmal focal vasodilatation. JAMA 1965; 191:691-694.
45. Medina JL, Diamond S: The clinical link between migraine and cluster headache. *Arch Neurol* 1977; 34:470-472.

2
Classification of Cluster Headache: Clinical Features of Episodic Cluster Headache

ROBERT S. KUNKEL

Cluster headache generally is less variable in its clinical presentation than the more frequently occurring migraine and muscle contraction headaches. There are, however, specific varieties of cluster headache which have been recognized and a classification of cluster headache has been generally accepted.

The acute episodic cluster headache is by far the most frequent pattern. Approximately 85% to 90% of patients with cluster headache have this form. Each individual headache is an attack while a series of attacks lasting several weeks or months forms a "cluster." The clinical presentation of those with acute episodic cluster headahces is discussed in detail in this chapter.

A small number of persons with very typical cluster type headache do not have remissions and are thus classified as having chronic cluster headache. Ekbom defined one as having chronic cluster headache if there were two or more headaches present each week for at least two years.[1] Others have used a criterion of two headaches a week for one year without a remission being present.[2] There are a few patients that have one or two weeks a year free of headaches who by these definitions are not "chronic cluster." About 10 to 15% of persons with cluster headache fall into the chronic category. A higher percentage of persons with chronic variety would probably be seen in various headache clinics. Chronic cluster headache was present in 15% of 435 patients recently reviewd by the author. Most patients with chronic cluster headache do not have several attacks a day and often have occasional headache free days whereas this is unusual in persons during the acute episodic cluster attack. Headache attacks usually occur daily in the acute episodic type; one to six attacks may hit in 24 hours.

Chronic cluster headache can further be categorized as a primary chronic form in which the patient has never had the acute episodic variety with remissions, or as a secondary chronic headache when acute episodic clusters have occurred in the past. A small number of patients will have chronic cluster headache for many years following which they will have a few years of remission only to have another reoccurrence of the chronic form. The sufferers with chronic cluster headache are by definition treatment failures in that a remission has not occurred either spontaneously or with medical therapy. Rarely, a chronic cluster pattern will evolve into an episodic form. About two thirds of the chronic cluster patients fall into the primary chronic category.

Cluster variants, or what may be known as atypical cluster headaches, refers to attacks of pain which seem to fall into a cluster pattern or which present with some of the features of the typical cluster attack but cannot be diagnosed as cluster headache. Cluster migraine is a headache which is migrainous by description but which has a clustering pattern. Chronic paroxysmal hemicrania, first described by Sjaastad, is felt to be a variant of cluster headache.[3,4] Typical cluster attacks and tic douloureux occasionally may occur in the same patient. Rarely typical tic type pains are accompanied by increased parasympathetic activity such as is common in cluster attacks.

In a detailed study of a group of cluster patients, Ekbom described upper and lower forms of cluster headaches.[1] The upper syndrome pain usually involves the eye, temple, forehead, and occipital area and is felt to be due to involvement of the external carotid system. Pain in the lower syndrome usually occurs in the forehead, temple, teeth, maxillary, and/or mandibular areas. This is felt to be due primarily to involvement of the internal carotid artery system. Although the upper and lower syndromes of cluster headache are usually not used when making a diagnosis or categorizing an attack, it should be noted that the pain in cluster headache attacks, though usually centered around the eye, can be quite widespread throughout the head, face and neck.

CLINICAL FEATURES OF EPISODIC CLUSTER HEADACHE

Cluster headache is an ailment predominantly of males. Just about 87 percent of my cluster patients are males.

Pain is the most striking symptom of the cluster attack. It is felt by most to be just about the most severe pain man can endure. Fortunately, the painful attack is of relatively short duration, rarely lasting more than two hours and it often lasts less than 30 minutes. Occasionally during a cluster with short attacks of pain, a long episode lasting several hours may occur. There is usually no aura present though some may feel a sensation in the upper nasal area at the onset of the attack. Visual symptoms such as are seen in the aura of the classic migraine attack are distinctly rare. The attack reaches its peak intensity in a few minutes. The pain may leave abruptly or may gradually lessen as the attack ceases. The intensity of the pain is so great that the victim usually jumps up and begins pacing the floor. He may perform calisthenics or other vigorous exercise. It is not unusual for patients to hit their head on the wall or the floor and stay in constant motion until the pain eases. A rare patient may be more comfortable lying still. These attacks, which may occur several times a day, often hit with striking regularity at the same time each day and often will occur in the early morning hours, one to two hours after retiring. I have had patients who changed shifts to work the midnight shift hoping to avoid the attack at night, but it then hit shortly after they retired in the morning.

The character of pain is described by the victim in various terms. It is rarely a pulsatile throbbing type of pain so typical of that experienced by the migraineur. The pain is usually steady and boring though it may be of a burning quality and at times will be described as sharp and stabbing. The feeling of a "hot poker in the eye" is a common description.

It is almost always centered around the eye. Most often the pain seems to be behind the eye giving the sensation that the eye is being pushed forward. Although centered around the orbit, the pain may be quite widespread occurring in the occiput, temple, frontal, or facial areas. Tenseness or tightness in the neck is commonly described. This may precede the severe orbital pain or may be more noticible as the pain eases. Radiation of the pain into the teeth of the upper and lower jaw is not uncommon and frequently teeth have been pulled in hopes of removing the source of the pain.

The cluster headache pain is essentially a unilateral pain. I can only recall one patient who had bilateral pains hitting during the same attack. The attacks of pain may shift from one side to another during the course of a cluster but it is much more common for the pain to remain on one side during a particular cluster. The pain may hit on the other side of the head when the next cluster arrives.

In contradistinction to the migraineur, the cluster victim rarely is nauseated. Vomiting is even more unusual. Though a study by Lance and Anthony found nausea or vomiting in about 50% of their cluster headache patients, I don't feel that these symptoms are that common.[5] Other common migraine symptoms such as photophobia and phonophobia may occur, but are distinctly less frequent than in migraine. Unilateral facial sweating is said to be a common occurrence during the attack although I am not impressed that it occurs very often.

Facial flushing may be present during the attack and is undoubtedly the reason for the condition having been called at one time "red migraine." The presence of facial flushing has recently been disputed.[6] The superficial temporal artery is often dilated and prominent during an attack. The artery and surrounding tissue may be quite tender to touch. Tenderness and soreness may be evident in the area between attacks of pain. Occasionally superficial scalp veins will be quite prominent during an attack.

Nasal congestion is frequently present during the attack on the ipsilateral side. Typically the congestion lessens along with the onset of some rinhorrhea as the pain eases. Some patients will note a burning in the nostril prior to the onset of the attack. Because of the nasal symptoms, allergies and sinus disease are often blamed for causing this particular headache. Many cluster patients get treated for recurrent sinus infections whenever a cluster hits.

The eye, which seems to be the focus of the pain in this condition, demonstrates several abnormalities in many cases. Since so few cluster attacks are actually observed by medical personnel, the incidence of eye signs is not accurately known. I suspect that they occur more often than is realized. Conjunctival infection with tearing of the affected eye probably occurs in 80% to 90% of attacks and usually, though not always, is present in association with nasal congestion and/or rhinorrhea.

Miosis with or without ptosis has been reported to occur in 15.5% and 18.3% of persons during a cluster attack.[1,7] In my experience, miosis is quite common if looked for specifically. It may remain after the attack of pain subsides. It may even remain after a cluster remits. Vision, though at times blurred is usually unaffected by the attack. Visual aberrations commonly seen in the classic

I.	Acute episodic cluster headache
II.	Chronic cluster headache
	A. Primary
	B. Secondary
III.	Cluster headache variants (atypical cluster)
	A. Cluster migraine
	B. Chronic paroxysmal hemicrania
	C. Cluster-tic
	D. Cluster-vertigo

Figure 1   Classification of Cluster Headache

migraine attacks rarely occur in the cluster patient. Ptosis and peri-orbital edema are not uncommon signs accompanying the attack.

Bradycardia may occur during the attack of cluster headache.[8,9] Blood pressure has been found to be increased along with the slowing of the pulse rate. Induced attacks of cluster headache also have shown P-wave changes.[9] These cardiovascular manifestations are probably due to increased parasympathetic activity causing increased vagal tone. The true incidence of these cardiovascular changes in unknown.

The person presenting with acute episodic cluster headache presents many striking clinical symptoms. The possible mechanism for these symptoms is discussed in detail by others in this volume.

REFERENCES

1. Ekbom K: A clinical comparison of cluster headache and migraine. *Acta Neurol Scand* 1970; 46(suppl 41):1-48.
2. Kunkel RS, Dohn DJ: Surgical treatment of chronic migrainous neuralgia. *Cleve Clin Q* 1974; 41:189-192.
3. Sjaastad O, and Dale I: A new clinical headache entity "Chronic Paroxysmal Hemicrania." *Acta Neurol Scand* 1976; 54:140-159.
4. Sjaastad O: So-called "vascular headache of the migraine type": One or more nosological entities? *Acta Neurol Scand* 1976; 454:125-139.
5. Lance JW, and Anthony M: Migrainous neuralgia or cluster headache. *J Neurol Sci* 1971; 13:401-414.
6. Ekbom K, and Kudrow L: Facial flush in cluster (editorial). *Headache* 1979; 19:47.
7. Kunkle EC, and Anderson WB: Dual mechanisms of eye signs of headache in cluster pattern. *Tr Am Neurol* 1960; 85:75-79.

8. Jacobson LB: Cluster headache: A rare cause of bradycardia. *Headache* 1969; 8:159-161.
9. Ekbom K: Heart rate, blood pressure and electrocardiographic changes during provoked attacks of cluster headache. *Acta Neurol Scand* 1970; 46:215-224.

3
Variants of Cluster Headache

SEYMOUR DIAMOND

CHRONIC CLUSTER HEADACHE

Cluster headache is a condition characterized by periods of frequent headaches alternating with headache-free periods. However, five to ten percent who experience attacks which are so typical of cluster (excruciating unilateral boring or burning pain located around the orbit or temple associated with unilateral autonomic symptoms) have extremely infrequent or possibly no periods of remission. These patients suffer from a variant of cluster known most commonly as "chronic cluster headache," or referred to as "chronic migrainous neuralgia" by authors who consider the first name a contradiction in terms.[1] Some of the patients with this syndrome have a history of more typically clustered headaches before the onset of the chronic pattern, and their disorder is termed *secondary* chronic cluster headache; those with no previous classical history are said to have the *primary* form.

Chronic cluster headaches were first recorded in 1947 by Ekbom[2] who noted chronic and periodic attacks occurring in the same patient. Between 1947 and 1969, several other authors described chronic cluster headaches in their patients.[3-5] In 1971 Ekbom[6] finally delineated a specific syndrome, termed "chronic cluster headache" and established criteria for inclusion in the syndrome of at least two headaches every week for one or more years.

There are several other features besides lack of periodicity which distinguish chronic cluster from episodic cluster: (1) an older age of onset in the chronic form (average age of onset, early 40s) as compared to episodic form (average age of onset, early 30s), (2) a different male to female ratio (6.3 to 1 in chronic, 4.8 to 1 in episodic cluster, [7] (3) increased headache frequency in chronic form, and (4) decreased responsiveness to the usual prophylactic medications, ergotamines, steroids, and methysergide[8] (although methysergide can ameliorate this condition temporarily, the serious side effects of long-term therapy preclude its consideration for treatment of this chronic disorder)[1] Such distinguishing characteristics as these suggest that the chronic form of cluster may actually be a separate disease entity.

At the time of his delineation of the chronic cluster syndrome, Ekbom reported results of treatment of five cluster patients (three chronic, two episodic) with lithium, chosen because of similarities between cluster headaches and manic-depressive illness.[2] The chronic patients showed dramatic results with exacerbation as soon as the drug was withdrawn, while episodic patients responded less dramatically.

Several other investigators have confirmed lithium's efficacy in chronic cluster with trials showing improvement in 75% to 100% of patients.[7,9-11] Long-term studies have demonstrated continued improvement up to 32 weeks in some patients.[8] However, tolerance has developed after eight months, although the pattern then seemed to change to episodic cluster.[10] Those patients who responded had dramatic results within the first two weeks of therapy.[7] Improvement in primary and secondary cluster patients was similar. However, all but one author[9] found lithium to be more efficacious in chronic than episodic cluster. Lithium did not appear to prevent alcohol-induced cluster attacks.[8] Side effects occurred in 25% to 85% of patients but were usually mild: tremors, weakness, lethargy, mild confusion, abdominal discomfort, diarrhea, lightheadedness, and insomnia.[12,8] Very few patients had to be withdrawn from studies because of side effects. The usual dose of lithium used was 300 mg three times daily, but authors titrated the dose to a serum level varying from 0.2 to 1.2 mEq/L.

The mechanism of action of lithium carbonate has not been elucidated. However, several theories have been proposed. Since lithium affects amine metabolism[13] and the potassium and sodium levels in various regions of the brain, Ekbom has speculated that specific actions of lithium in the central nervous system may help ameliorate

cluster.[10] A decrease in monoamine oxidase (MAO) activity has been shown during cluster attacks,[14] and it is postulated that lithium's effect of increasing platelet MAO activity may help prevent cluster headaches by stabilizing MAO levels.[15] Klimek proposes a possible mechanism of action through lithium's inhibitory effect on acetylcholine since symptoms of cholinergic hyperfunction (lacrimation, conjunctival injection, rhinorrhea) are observed in cluster attacks.[9]

One of the newest theories of lithium action in chronic cluster involves its effects on REM sleep. Mendel and Chernik[16] and Kupfer[17] have reported a decrease in mean REM frequency and increased latency of the first REM sleep following lithium administration. Since chronic cluster attacks occur with remarkable regularity at night and are associated with REM sleep,[18] this action of lithium may be linked to its efficacy in chronic cluster, and indeed, lithium has been shown to delay the timing of cluster attacks until morning. Whatever the mechanism of action, lithium's efficacy in cluster appears to be independent of its antidepressant effects.

In conclusion, chronic cluster headache is a recently discovered clinical syndrome characterized by identical symptoms of episodic cluster headache occurring chronically. The demographic features, as well as the therapeutic responsiveness of these periodic and chronic cluster patient populations, are sufficiently distinct to suggest that they represent separate syndromes. Chronic cluster headache patients have shown a good response to lithium, and in the future this drug may gain universal acceptance as the medication of choice in the prophylaxis of this syndrome.

CYCLIC MIGRAINE

The headaches characteristically occur in groups separated by periods free, or relatively free, of headache. The duration of the cycles varies between two and twenty weeks, and the cycle frequency ranges between one and twelve per year, with an average of five per year. During the cycles, the headaches occur at the rate of one to seven per week, with an average of 4.8 per week. A frequent symptom during the cycle is a constant low-intensity, unilateral, or bilateral headache between the migraine attacks.

Although this headache bears some similarities to cluster headache, many differences can be pointed out: (1) Cyclic migraine is long lasting, with an average duration of 25.5 hours, (2) the location of cyclical migraine is either bilateral or may occur on either side in patients with unilateral headache, and (3) in cyclical migraine, auras of scintillating scotomas or other focal neurological symptoms are frequent.

The cyclical nature of this headache, and its response to lithium carbonate, resembles manic-depressive illness. The cycles, however, are much shorter than in manic-depressive illness, and the severity of the mood change is also much less than in manic-depressive illness. Nevertheless, a similar cyclical biochemical phenomena may be involved in both conditions.

To diagnose this condition, the following criteria should be met: (1) the patient should have classical or nonclassical migraine, (2) the headaches should occur in cycles lasting two or more weeks, (3) during the cycle the patient should have clearly separated multiple headache attacks, and (4) there should be evidence of at least two previous cycles. The reason for the second and third criteria is that some migraines may last as long as one week and, therefore, one may confuse a recurrent, prolonged migraine with a cyclical migraine.

Lithium carbonate seems to be the drug of choice for therapy in this condition because of the small dosage needed and the prompt response. All patients with cyclical migraine should be tried on lighium carbonate for about two weeks. If the patient responds, he should continue to take lithium carbonate for at least one month longer than the anticipated duration of the headache cycle. The usual precautions in the use of lithium carbonate should be taken.

THE SPECTRUM OF A NEW CLUSTER HEADACHE VARIANT SYNDROME AND ITS RESPONSE TO INDOMETHACIN

The syndrome consists of three symptoms occurring in different patients in various combinations: (1) atypical cluster headaches, (2) multiple jabs, and (3) background vascular headaches. Atypical cluster headaches are chronic headaches that, like cluster headaches, occur several times per day. They are considered atypical because of their location, duration and /or frequent shifting and/or frequency. These headaches are often accompanied by multiple jabs and associated with background vascular headaches. Multiple jabs are sharp pains of variable severity and location that last for a few seconds and occur several times every day or almost daily. Background vascular headache is a continuous, often unilateral headache of variable severity which is usually throbbing or becomes throbbing during exertion.

We studied 54 patients between the ages of 14 and 78 (average = 40.5 years). Twenty-eight were female and twenty-six were male. Forty-six of the 54 patients had atypical cluster headaches, 28 patients had background vascular headaches and 20 patients had multiple jabs. Forty-five patients (83%) responded to indomethacin. All nine patients who failed to respond to indomethacin were depressed. These nine patients responded well to tricyclic antidepressants.

CHRONIC PAROXYSMAL HEMICRANIA

First described in 1974 by Sjaastad and Ade,[19,20] chronic paroxysmal hemicrania is a rare variant of cluster headache. It is characterized by the frequent, daily (chronic) occurrence of excruciating unilateral and same-sided headache attacks (hemicrania) lasting 15 to 30 minutes (paroxysmal) in most cases, and primarily localized to the temporal region. The headaches are usually associated with autonomic symptoms including ipsilateral tearing, conjunctival injection, nasal stuffiness or rhinorrhea, Horner's syndrome, and extrasystoles or bradycardia.

It appears that patients first pass through a pre-CPH stage during which their headaches resemble tension headache, common migraine, or are a less severe or less frequent version of a typical CPH attack. This pre-CPH stage may last for many years before the more classical headache pattern of CPH begins, in all cases at greater than twenty years of age. As might be expected, recognition of this syndrome while the patient is still in the pre-CPH stage is extremely difficult and most patients are seen by a multitude of specialists before they are correctly diagnosed and treated.

Indomethacin dramatically prevents the headache attacks, with results apparent as early as several hours after the first dose. The usual starting dose is 25 to 50 mg PO TID and the final dose varies between 12.5 to 25 mg PO QID. If the patient begins treatment while still in the pre-CPH stage, the indomethacin dose may be tapered and eventually discontinued without recurrence of the headaches. However, once the true CPH attack pattern has ensued, treatment must be continued on a chronic basis, or symptoms will resume within a very short time.

CPH differs from classical or chronic cluster headaches in several respects which may aid in diagnosis.

1. The individual attacks are of shorter duration, usually 15 to 30 minutes, but occur with a much greater maximum frequency,

more than 15 in 24 hours. They occur daily with no night preponderance.

2. Some patients may mechanically precipitate attacks by bending forward or turning their head toward the affected side.

3. There is a clear female predominance in CPH.

4. An association between pregnancy and CPH exists, as evidenced by the amelioration of the severity and frequency of attacks during pregnancy. In some patients, the onset of headache attacks occurs immediately after delivery.

5. Corneal indentation pulses markedly increase in amplitude at the onset of an attack.[21]

6. Essential to the diagnosis of CPH is a complete response to indomethacin, whereas the effect of this drug on cluster headache is variable.

An increasing number of case reports of chronic paroxysmal hemicrania are appearing in the literature as it becomes a more clearly defined disease entity.[22] Our ability to so effectively treat this incapacitating disorder of frequent excruciating headaches places paramount importance on our ability to recognize the symptoms, and it rewards our patients and ourselves handsomely when we are able to make this diagnosis.

CLUSTER MIGRAINE HEADACHES

Most authors believe that both cluster and migraine headaches are vascular in origin, but they still do not agree whether to consider cluster headaches a variant of migraine[23-25] or a completely different disorder.[26-29] The authors who link these disorders emphasize their similarities and those who separate them stress the differences.

The relationship between migraine and cluster headaches can be strengthened by noting some patients whose headaches present features common to both cephalagias. These patients represent a clinical link between the disorders and strongly suggest that cluster and migraine headaches are part of the spectrum of the same entity.

Transient visual symptoms in the form of hemianoptic, quandrantic, or other scotomata preceding headache have been considered to be pathognomonic of classical migraine with rare exceptions.[30,31] Sutherland and Eadie[32] described a patient who on one occasion had visual scintillations prior to a cluster headache, and Duvoisin et al[33] reported a patient with cluster headaches who had prodromic scotomata.

The presence of contralateral sensory and motor symptoms preceding or accompanying migraine is a common finding[34] that has been attributed to constriction of intracerebral arteries.[35] Contralateral focal symptoms, as well as ipsilateral visual disturbances, might be expected with cluster headaches because of the presence of vasoconstriction of the internal carotid artery in some patients during cluster headaches.[36] Contralateral paresthesias, to our knowledge, have only been described in two patients[32] and motor symptoms have only been observed by Sutherland and Eadie[32] and Sjaastad et al,[37] in two patients who had twitching of the extremities contralateral to their headaches. However, ipsilateral blurring of vision in cluster headache is common and it has been discounted as due to the tearing that accompanies the headache; however, dimness without lacrimation has been observed by Lance and Anthony.[38]

Cluster headache characteristically occurs in groups of attacks for several weeks followed by long free periods. However, this pattern only occurs in 93% of the patients with cluster headaches,[28] and it is not pathognomonic for them. Sacks[39] described a 55-year-old patient who had five or six weeks of bouts of common migraine headaches every year.

Certain pathophysiological and biochemical data have been presented by Ekbom[40] as significant supporting evidence for the differentiation of cluster and migraine headaches as distinct entities. Horven et al[41] did dynamic tonometry during headaches and demonstrated that, in contrast to migraine, there was increase in the intraocular pressure synchronous with the pulse in cluster headache. They believed that this effect was caused by pulsatile changes in the intraocular volume due to vasodilation of the choroidal vessels. These findings correlated well with the dilation of the ophthalmic artery noted in the angiograms of patients during cluster headaches.[36] Thermography has shown the presence of hypothermic islands in the periorbital skin in 85% of patients with cluster headaches, but in only 2% of migrainous patients.[42] These hypothermic spots are frequently located in areas of the skin supplied by branches of the internal carotid arteries. Obviously, these pathophysiological studies do not provide an etiologic differentiation and only show that during the headache phase migraine involves mainly the external carotid circulation, and cluster headaches, the internal carotid circulation. Certain biochemical changes have been claimed to be specific for each of these headaches. Platelet serotonin level was found to be reduced during the pain phase of migraine and histamine level was found to be increased during cluster headache.[43] However, Wilkinson[44] and Ziegler et al[45] did not find any consistent change in serotonin level during migraine. Furthermore, Anthony and Lance[43] showed a notable elevation of histamine level during migraine headaches, but not so pronounced as in cluster headaches. The difference in the level elevation of these vasoactive substances may represent different degrees of the same phenomenon occurring in both headaches. Therefore, pathophysiological and biochemical changes have not conclusively established a difference between cluster and migraine headaches, and clinical symptoms provide the basis for classifying these headaches. This is not always simple, since manifestations that have been considered almost pathognomonic for migraine have also occurred with cluster headaches, and the characteristic grouping of headaches in clusters occurs with migraine.

REFERENCES

1. Pearce JM: Chronic migrainous neuralgia: A variant of cluster headache. *Brain* 1980; 103:149-159.
2. Ekbom, KA: Ergotamine tartrate orally in Horton's "histaminic cephalgia": a new method of treatment. *Acta Psychiatr Neurol* 1947; 46 (suppl): 105-113.
3. Symonds C: A particular variety of headaches. *Brain* 1956; 79:217-232.
4. Rooke ED, Rushton JG, Peters GA: Vasodilating headaches: A suggestive classification and results of prophylactic treatment with UML 491 (methysergide). *Proc Staff Meet Mayo Clin* 1962; 37:433.
5. McArdle MJ: Variants of migraine. in Cummings JN (ed): *Background to Migraine: Second International Symposium.* London, Heinemann, 1969, pp 3-4.
6. Ekbom K, De Fine OB: Chronic migrainous neuralgia—diagnostic and therapeutic aspects. *Headache* 1971; 11:97-101.
7. Kudrow L: *Cluster Headache.* Oxford, Oxford University Press, 1980, pp 12-14.
8. Kudrow L: Lithium prophylaxis for chronic cluster headaches. *Headache* 1977; 17:15-18.
9. Klimek A, Szulc-Kuberska J, Kawiorski S: Lithium therapy in cluster headache. *Eur Neurol* 1979; 18:267-268.
10. Ekbom K: Lithium for cluster headache: Literature review. *Headache* 1981; 21:132-139.
11. Matthew NT: Clinical subtypes of cluster headache and response to lithium therapy. *Headache* 1978; 18:26-30.
12. Matthew NT: Lithium therapy in cluster headache. *Headache* 1977; 17: 15-18.
13. Corrodi H, Fuxe K, Hokfelt T, Shou M: The effect of lithium on cerebral monoamine neurons. *Psychopharmacologia* 1967; 11:345-353.
14. Bockar F, Roth R, Heninger G: Increased human platelet monoamine oxidase activity during lithium carbonate therapy. *Life Sci* 1974; 15:2109-2118.

15. Lieb J, Zeff A: Lithium treatment of chronic cluster headaches. *Br J Psychiat* 1978; 133:556-558.
16. Mendels J, Chernik DA: The effect of lithium carbonate on the sleep of depressed patients. *Int Pharmaco-Psychiat* 1978; 8:184-192.
17. Kupfer DJ, Wyatt RJ, Greenspan K, Scott J, Snyder F: Lithium carbonate and sleep in affective illness. *Arch Gen Psychiat* 1970; 23:35-40.
18. Ekbom K: Lithium in the treatment of chronic cluster headache. *Headache* 1977; 17:39-40.
19. Sjaastad, O, Dale I: Evidence for a new (?) treatable headache entity: A preliminary report *Headache* 1974; 14:105-108.
20. Sjaastad O, Dale I: A new (?) clinical headache entity: A preliminary report. *Headache* 1974; 14:105-108.
21. Sjaastad O, Egge K, Horven I, et al: Chronic paroxysmal hemicrania: Mechanical precipitation of attacks. *Headache* 1979; 19(1):31-36.
22. Price RW, Posner JB: Chronic paroxysmal hemicrania: A disabling headache syndrome responding to indomethacin. *Ann Neur* 1978; 3:184-184.
23. Wolff HG: *Headache and Other Head Pain*, ed 2. New York, Oxford University Press, 1963.
24. Friedman AP: The migraine syndrome. *Bull NY Acad Med* 1968; 44:45-62.
25. Bickerstaff ER: The periodic migrainous neuralgia of Wilfred Harris. *Lancet* 1959; 1:1069-1071.
26. Horton BT, McLean AR, Craig W: A new syndrome of vascular headache: Results of treatment with histamine: Preliminary reports. *Proc Staff Meet Mayo Clin* 1939; 14:257-260.
27. Robinson BW: Histaminic cephalagia. *Medicine* 1958; 37:161-180.
28. Ekbom K: A clinical comparison of cluster headache and migraine. *Acta Neurol Scand* 1970; 41(suppl):1-48.
29. Sjaastad O: So-called "vascular headache of the migraine type": One or more nosological entities? *Acta Neurol Scand* 1976; 54:125-139.
30. Fisher CM: Some neuro-ophthalmological observations. *J. Neurol Neurosurg Psychiatry* 1967; 30:383-392.
31. Aring CD: The migrainous scintillating scotoma *JAMA* 1972; 220:519-522.
32. Sutherland M, Eadie MJ: Cluster headache. *Res Clin Stud Headache* 3:92-125, 1972.
33. Duvoisin RC, Parker GW, Kenoyer WL: The cluster headache. *Arch Intern Med* 1961; 108:711-716.
34. Carroll JD: Migraine, its variants, differential diagnosis and treatment. *Res Clin Stud Headache* 1967; 1:46-61.
35. Dalessio DJ: *Wolff's Headache and Other Head Pain.* New York, Oxford University Press, 1972.
36. Ekbom K, Greitz T: Carotid angiography in cluster headache. *Acta Radiol Diagn* 1970; 20:177-186.
37. Sjaastad O, Horven I, Vennerod AM: A new headache syndrome; Headache resembling cluster headache (Horton's headache), with recurring bouts of homolateral retrabulbar neuritis partial factor XII deficiency, bleeding tendency and a heterolateral convulsive episode. *Headache* 1976; 16:4-10.
38. Lance JW, Anthony M: Migrainous neuralgia or cluster headache. *J Neurol Sci* 1971; 13:401-414.

39. Sacks OW: *Migraine: The Evaluation of a Common Disorder*. New York, University of California Press, 1970.

40. Ekbom K: Clinical aspects of cluster headache. *Headache* 1974; 13:176-180.

41. Horven I, Nornes H, Sjaastad O: Different corneal indentation pulse pattern in cluster headache and migraine. *Neurology* 1972; 22:92-98.

42. Friedman AP, Wood EH, Rowan AS, et al: Observations on vascular headache of the migraine type, in Cumings JN (ed): *Background to Migraine: Fifth Migraine Symposium*. New York, Springer-Verlag, 1973, pp 1-17.

43. Anthony M, Lance JW: Histamine and serotonin in cluster headache. *Arch Neurol* 25:225-231, 1971.

44. Wilkinson M: Some aspects of the role of tyramine in the production of headache, in Diamond S, Dalessio DJ, Graham JR, et al (eds): *Vasoactive Substances Relevant to Migraine*. Springfield, IL, Charles C. Thomas Publisher, 1975, pp. 86-89.

45. Ziegler DK, Stephenson HR, Ward DF: Migraine, tyramine and blood serotonin. *Headache* 1976; 16:53-57.

4
Nonheadache Disorders and Characteristics of Cluster Headache Patients

JOEL R. SAPER

Cluster headache stands far and above most other headache conditions in its distinctive stereotypical clinical presentation. The incidence of cluster headache is estimated at 1% or less.[1] In 1969 and later in 1972[2,3], Graham described a constellation of somatic and personality traits believed to characterize many, if not most, cluster headache patients. These astute observations, together with earlier ones, prompted further consideration of the physical features, accompanying medical disorders, and psychological profiles of patients with cluster headache.[1,4-16] This paper reviews the current understanding of the nonheadache features and medical conditions of cluster headache patients. When possible, attention will be paid to any existing differences between chronic and episodic subtypes.

GENERAL PHYSICAL FEATURES

Facial Features

Graham[2,3] first noted that many cluster headache patients had similar facial appearance, featuring a ruddy complexion and multi-furrowed and thick skin. Deep furrows in the forehead, assymetrical vertical creases at the glabella, and prominent nasal labial folds were evident. The skull was broad and the chin square and often "upholstered." Pitted, coarse skin similar to an orange peel was noted. This leonized appearance typified many cluster headache men and some cluster headache women. Ekbom and Greitz[17] confirmed the presence of widened skulls in cluster headache patients, including women.

The leonized features were not likely to be prominent in earlier life, but developed as patients became older. Initially, Graham postulated that this facial appearance was possibly related to elevated serotonin and bradykinin levels, because of the similarity between the cluster headache facies and some patients with carcinoid syndrome. Lance and Anthony[18], however, were not able to confirm elevations of these substances. The similarity between the typical facies of a cluster headache patient and that seen in many chronic alcoholics was also noted.[0]

Kudrow[5] suggested that the facial features in male cluster headache patients resulted from excessive smoking and drinking. He noted that these habits were likely to induce the skin changes in cluster headache patients and noncluster headache individuals who drank and smoked excessively.[19]

Height

Kudrow[1,5] suggested that male cluster headache patients, in addition to having a particular facial appearance, were likely to demonstrate other similar physical traits. In a study of 240 cluster headache males, a statistically significant increase in height as compared to controls and to average American males was noted. Schele et al[8] also noted that cluster males were taller than noncluster males from the same geographic region. Saper et al[16], studying 155 cluster headache patients identified no statistically significant difference in height among male and female patients as compared to controls.

Weight

To date, no significant differences in weight have been noted between cluster headache patients and noncluster headache persons.[1,16]

Eye Color

Kudrow[1,5] found a significantly higher incidence of hazel eye color in the cluster headache group when compared to controls, 38% and 9% respectively. An incidence of 8% hazel eye color is documented in the general population.[20]

Saper et al[16] could not demonstrate a statistically significant difference with regard to eye color between the *total* cluster headache group and that of controls. However, a significant increase in hazel colored eyes in the chronic subtype of cluster headache, both males and females, was found when measured against episodie (classic) cluster headache (males and females) and controls.

PSYCHOLOGICAL CHARACTERISTICS

Graham[3] portrayed cluster headache males as rugged in stature, possessing athletic prowess, aggressive, and masculine. They were heavier drinkers and smokers than migraine controls (see below) and were ambitious, hard working, demonstrating a strong sense of upward mobility, perhaps driving themselves to exhaustion and headaches. Beneath the viril exterior, however, Graham described marked dependency needs, a reluctance to divulge true feelings, intense feelings of anger, insecurity, and guilt. Cluster headache males were often led and represented by their wives, and Graham likened this to a powerful mouse pulling a red wagon in which was proudly perched Leo the Lion.

Under pressure, cluster patients had a tendency toward "a peculiar form of hysterical behavior." The pacing, yelling, and head banging behavior frequently seen during painful events[3] (see below) might, it was suggested, reflect this hysterical tendency. The presence of depression, maybe a result of ambivalence toward parental dominance or strained father–son relationships, was also common. Cluster headache patients did not do well in psychotherapeutic settings.

Steinhilber et al[11], focusing on perfectionist, rigid, and approval seeking behavior described earlier by Friedman et al[13] studied the Minnesota Multiphasic Personality Inventory (MMPI) of 50 cluster headache patients. Although he found that high scores on hypochondriasis and hysteria scales, and lower scores on depression scales were common, the findings were not unlike "other headache groups."

Kudrow[1,5,7] suggested that the cluster headache population was typified by reserved, rigid, detached, and self-critical personalities. Patients tended to be conscientious, persistent, staid, and moralistic. Kudrow noted that cluster headache individuals were self-sufficient, resourceful, socially precise, compulsive, tense, and easily frustrated. Studying MMPI results of 41 patients with cluster headache Kudrow and Sutkus[7] found that migraine and cluster headache groups scored similarly on all scales, showing no conversion "V" configuration.

However, when cluster headache males were compared to nonheadache controls, higher hypochondriasis, hysteria, and depression scores were noted, although no value reached a "T" score of 65, above which is generally considered abnormal. When averaged for a single value for psychopathology, the Kudrow studies suggested that cluster headache patients did not differ significantly from that of controls.

Rogado et al[12], studying 50 cluster headache patients and matched migraine controls, showed that cluster patients had higher scores than controls on hysteria and hypochondriasis, but did not differ from controls for depression. Obsessive-compulsive (psychasthenia) tendencies were also higher in cluster headache patients than in controls, a finding that was not substantiated by the study of Kudrow and Sutkus.[7]

Saper et al,[16] studying 101 cluster headache patients (77 males, 24 females), and 62 age-sex matched controls, observed that 41% of cluster headache patients experienced suicidal ideation during a headache which compared to only 10% of controls, a difference which reached statistical significance. The female chronic cluster headache subtype seemed most likely to harbor suicidal thoughts during a headache. Few cluster headache patients admitted however, that suicidal planning had been undertaken. Only 7% identified suicidal thoughts during nonheadache periods.

Saper et al[16] also noted that cluster headache patients, when compared to noncluster headache controls, were statistically more likely to pound their fists, yell, and pace than were noncluster headache controls, who preferred to sleep during their attacks. Twenty-five percent of male and female cluster headache patients pounded their fists and yelled during a headache, while over half paced during an attack.

OCCUPATION

Kudrow[1] studied the occupations of 325 cluster headache males and compared these to 200 male controls, and demonstrated that occupational distribution in both groups was similar. No support was found to suggest that cluster headache males tended to select high pressure, responsibility oriented occupations.

Saper et al[16] studying four occupational categories (professional, white collar, blue collar, and "others") found male cluster headache patients, to a statistically significant degree, were more likely to have professional occupations than were noncluster headache males. This was not so in the female population.

HABITS

Smoking and Drinking

Graham[3] drew attention to the tendency for cluster headache patients to drink alcohol and smoke excessively. Kudrow[5], studying the smoking and drinking habits of cluster headache men and women with a mean age of 42, found that 94% of cluster headache patients smoked cigarettes, compared 63% of the noncluster headache control group, a statistically significant difference. In a later work[1], Kudrow again found that a greater percentage of cluster patients smoked than did controls, but a general decrease in the overall incidence of smoking since the 1974 study was noted.

Saper et al[16] in their 1981 study (detailed previously) found that 66% of cluster headache patients smoked cigarettes, compared to 17% of noncluster headache controls, a difference also reaching statistical significance. This tendency towards smoking crossed all cluster headache categories. Cluster headache patients smoked for a mean of 15 years prior to this study.

Kudrow[5] noted 91% of cluster headache patients drank alcohol, and 61% were considered moderate to excessive drinkers (moderate to excessive drinking was considered to be no less than three ounces of hard liquor or a 6 pack of beer or 12 ounces of wine per day). Sixty-five percent of controls drank alcohol, and only 20% were moderate to excessive in their intake.

Saper et al[16] found 61% of patients with cluster headache and 41% of noncluster headache controls to consume alcohol *at least* occasionally when not experiencing headaches. Thirty-six percent of cluster headache patients as compared to 13% of noncluster headache controls admitted to the consumption of alcohol daily, representing a statistically significant difference. At least 21% of cluster headache males acknowledged that they were unable to give up alcohol even when experiencing headaches, which were characteristically alcohol sensitive. By contrast, cluster headache females did not drink during cluster headache periods, and all cluster headache women reported the ability to completely avoid alcohol consumption during headache bouts, despite 20% of cluster headache women acknowledging that between cluster periods they drank alcohol daily.

Gun Ownership

Based upon the bedside observation that hospitalized cluster headache patients were likely to have gun and hunting magazines on their night table and spoke of guns frequently, Saper et al[16] studied a Michigan population. They found that 71% of 77 male and 24% of 24 women cluster headache patients own guns, which compared to 60% of men and 15% of women in the age-sex matched control group of 62 patients, a difference that reached statistical significance in both groups. Many patients remarked that during bouts of cluster attacks, the guns were removed from the home by the spouse.

LABORATORY ABNORMALITIES

Hematocrit and Hemoglobin

Over half of patients with cluster headache were reported by Graham[4] to have hematocrit readings of 46% or over, with some reaching levels of 50%. Saper et al[16] also reported statistically higher hematocrit readings in cluster headache patients when compared to controls. Schele et al[8] reported normal hematocrit values in cluster headache patients.

Kudrow[5], studying a small group of cluster headache patients found that hemoglobin values were higher in the cluster population than in controls. In a subsequent survey[1] Kudrow did not find hemoglobin values elevated. Saper et al[16] also found normal values for hemoglobin.

White Blood Count

Cluster headache patients were noted by Saper et al[16] to exhibit a higher total white blood cell count than noncluster headache controls. Mean white count for cluster headache patients was 8,478, as compared to 6,500 for controls, a difference reaching statistical significance. Studying different cluster subtypes, it appeared that episodic cluster headache patients had a much higher white count than chronic cluster headache patients, and this difference seemed to account for the differences between cluster headache patients as a group and that of controls. (86% of cluster patients were evaluated during cluster periods.) Differential counts did not reveal abnormalities.

The importance of this difference in WBC determinations may be influenced by the retrospective recognition that many cluster headache patients of both episodic and chrnoic subtypes were or had recently been on lithium carbonate, known to provoke leukocytosis. Nonetheless, episodic cluster headache patients appear to have WBC elevations as compared to those with chronic cluster headache and controls.

Triglyceride Level

Graham[3] suggested that abnormal lipid patterns were present in 16 of 23 cluster headache patients, and Olesen[21] described several cases of essential hyperlipidemia. Saper et al[16] could not find significant differences between the total cluster group and noncluster headache populations in terms of triglyceride blood levels. However, chronic cluster headache males and females had a statistically significant increase in mean triglyceride levels when compared to male and females with episodic cluster headache, who had a significantly lower triglyceride reading than male and female controls.

Cholesterol readings and sedimentation rates did not differ between cluster headache populations and controls.[16]

FAMILY HISTORY OF HEADACHES

Graham[3] noted that 17% of cluster patient relatives (father, mother, and siblings) had migraine, and 6% had cluster headaches, numbers much higher than relatives of controls. He cited a previous study, which included aunts, uncles, and grandparents, similarly showing an increased incidence of migraine exceeding that found in the general population, although not higher than that found in the relatives of known migraine patients. Kudrow[1] considering available evidence[3,15,22] concluded that a positive family history of migraine among cluster headache patients varied between 15 and 21%, which was not much different than the incidence in the control population.

Kudrow found the incidence of cluster headache in family members of cluster headache patients ranged from 0%[15] to 4.7%[1]. In Kudrow's study, the incidence of cluster headache in parents of cluster headache patients ranged from 2% to 6%.

THE PRESENCE OF MIGRAINE IN CLUSTER
HEADACHE PATIENTS

Ekbom[22,23] suggested that between 2.9% and 3.1% of cluster headache patients also had migraine. Graham[3] found that 27% of cluster headache patients had a history of migraine. In a study by Lance and Anthony[18] 6.7% of cluster headache patients were noted to have migraine. Kudrow[6] proposed that migraine occurred in approximately 17% of cluster headache patients, an incidence midway between the 27% noted by Graham and the 6.7% noted by Anthony and Lance. Kudrow noted, however, a dramatic increase in the incidence of migraine in women with cluster headache, as compared to an incidence in males similar to that expected for males in general.[1]

MEDICAL DISORDERS IN CLUSTER HEADACHE PATIENTS

Peptic Ulcer Disease

Several earlier reports raised the possibility of an increased incidence of peptic ulcer disease in cluster headache patients.[24-27] In 1968 Ekbom and Kugelberg[28] reported an overall incidence of 13% of peptic ulcer in their patients with cluster headache. In a later study, Ekbom[29] studying 89 males with cluster headache identified an overall ulcer history in 17%. This compared to an ulcer incidence of between 20% and 22% reported by Graham.[2,3] Graham, like Horton,[24] suggested that high gastric acid secretion rates were present in many of these patients, approaching that seen in the Zollinger-Ellison syndrome.

Kudrow[6], studying 119 male and 21 female patients with cluster headache, found 21.2% of males had peptic ulcer disease, predominantly duodenal, as compared to 10.7% of male migraine controls. Peptic ulcer disease in cluster women was substantially higher than in migraine women controls. Both were above that estimated for women in the general population. A recent report by Kudrow[1] demonstrated results similar to the 1976 report, estimating the incidence of peptic ulcer to be approximately 19.7% in males.

Saper et al[16] was not able to show a statistically significant difference between cluster headache males with ulcer disease and male noncluster headache controls.

Hypertension

Kudrow[1,6] reported that the incidence of hypertension in cluster headache patients was less than that in controls, though not to a degree reaching statistical significance. Saper et al[16] noted a lower diastolic blood pressure in cluster headache patients as measured against controls, a difference reaching statistical significance. Systolic pressures, however, were not significantly different.

Coronary Artery Disease

Kudrow[6] noted that coronary artery disease seemed to be more common in cluster males but not to a statistically singificant degree, and none of the cluster headache women had any evidence of coronary artery disease among cluster headache patients. Saper et al[16] found that the incidence of a history of myocardial infarction in male cluster headache patients was substantially greater than in male controls, although like other studies the difference did not reach statistical significance.

Ekbom[10,29] identified a reduction in anginal attacks during cluster periods. Ekbom and Lindahl[10] demonstrated an elevation of threshold for angina pectoris induction during cluster periods, and suggested that alterations in vasoreactivity of cranial blood vessels occurred during cluster periods and remission, indirectly influencing cardiac function. Graham[30] described two patients who experienced remission of intermittent claudication only during spontaneous cluster attacks. He also noted that studies tended to measure younger age groups, and suggested that were cluster headache patients to be assessed for the incidence of coronary artery disease at an older age, an increased incidence would likely be identified.[31]

Several authors have reported the association of episodic bradycardia in the cluster headache population.[32-36]

Cancer

In a recent study, Kudrow[1] demonstrated a higher than expected incidence of cancer in cluster headache patients. In a study of 230 males, 3.5% had a current or past history of cancer, as compared to 0.3% of the general male population.

Other Disorders

Several other disorders have been identified in patients with cluster headache. Lance[15] reported nine out of 60 patients suffered from allergic disorders. Two had hives, two experienced asthma, and four suffered from hay fever. One patient had both asthma and hay fever. Two patients appeared to experience cluster headache bouts within two to four weeks after episodes of hay fever. One of these reported that as the hay fever became milder each year, the cluster bouts became longer and more intense.

Friedman and Mikropoulous[13] reported an allergy incidence in cluster headache patients of 12%, while Lance and Anthony[18] reported an incidence of 15%. Schele et al[8] noted a 22% incidence of allergic conditions in cluster headache patients, but did not feel that this reached statistical significance.

A history of head trauma has been reported in eight of 60 patients reported by Lance[15], and in four, the location of injury was possibly relevant to the ensuing cluster headache. Head trauma has also been reported by others.[13,37]

Kudrow[1] notes more than one-third of cluster headache males had tonsillectomies performed in childhood, and 16.5% had surgery for acute appendicitis. Herniorrhaphy took place in 7.4%, nasal surgery in 4.8%, and cervical or lumbar disc surgery in 3.9% of the cluster headache patients.

SUMMARY OF FINDINGS

The following represents this author's summary of current evidence on the nonheadache features of cluster headache patients.

1. A substantial number of cluster headache patients, including some women, demonstrate rugged, lined, and leonized facies, perhaps to a degree greater than that which would be expected by chance alone. In addition, studies support a higher than expected incidence of hazel or blue colored eyes in cluster headache patients, and this may be even more so in the chronic cluster headache subtype.

2. Cluster headache male patients *may* be somewhat taller as a group than controls, but reports are not in unanimous agreement. Weight differences have not been demonstrated.

3. The available evidence suggests that many cluster headache patients exhibit what has been characterized as hysterical behavior, particularly during headache attacks. Cluster headache patients may

have higher scores on hysteria and hypochondriasis scales of the MMPI than nonheadache controls, but not necessarily higher than noncluster headache controls. Suicide ideation during attacks seems evident in many cluster headache patients.

4. Both cluster headache males and females appear to have a substantially greater likelihood of excessive alcohol ingestion and smoking than controls.

5. The "rugged" character of many male and some female cluster headache patients may even extend to a greater tendency to own guns. Gun ownership and the violent/rage behavior during cluster headache attacks may perhaps reflect deeply repressed emotions as described by Graham.

6. Cluster headache patients may have higher hematocrit readings than controls, although studies disagree on this point. Hemoglobin values appear to be no different than in controls.

7. White blood count values *may* be elevated in cluster headache patients, particularly during cluster attacks. This tendency may be most evident in episodic subtypes as compared to chronic subtypes. That this finding is factitious, reflecting therapeutic interventions, cannot at this time be excluded.

8. Triglyceride levels may be higher in patients with cluster headache, particularly the chronic subtype, than in controls. Cholesterol readings appear no different in cluster headache than in controls.

9. Migraine may be more common in patients who also have cluster headache, particularly females, than in control groups.

10. Ulcer disease appears more likely to occur in cluster headache males and females than in the general population.

11. Cluster headache patients may have a lower incidence of hypertension than controls. In addition, cluster headache patients may as a group have somewhat lower readings than controls.

12. A trend toward a higher incidence of coronary artery disease is present, though not at this time reaching statistical significance. Were studies to assess an older cluster headache population and controls than is currently reflected, this trend might reach significance.

13. A higher incidence of cancer might be present in male cluster headache patients than in male controls; however, only one study to date has addressed this issue.

14. The relationship between cluster headache and allergy head trauma, and other illnesses is less clear and uncertain than it is on the previously mentioned disorders and characteristics.

CONCLUSIONS

Cluster headache patients appear prone to certain physical characteristics and a tendency toward particular illnesses, to smoke and drink excessively and have elevated lipid levels, and demonstrate certain personality features. Several of these such as leonized facial features, ulcer disease and coronary artery disease risk may actually reflect the consequences of excessive smoking and drinking. However, if valid, the higher incidence of hazel colored eyes, greater height, personality similarities, and the inclination to drink and smoke may indicate that cluster headache patients are biologically predisposed to a constellation of somatic, physical, and emotional characteristics, of which headache is perhaps the most dramatic. Excessive smoking and drinking may themselves be manifestations of this tendency, rather than playing an entirely causative role. Further studies, isolating these and other variables, are necessary in order to unravel the mystery of cluster headaches and those who suffer from them.

REFERENCES

1. Kudrow L: Cluster headache. Mechanisms and management. New York, Oxford University Press, 1980.
2. Graham JR: Cluster headache. Presentation, International Symposium on Headache, Chicago, IL, Oct 1969.
3. Graham JR: Cluster headache. *Headache* 1972; 11:175-185.
4. Graham JR, Rogado AZ, Rahman M, et al: Dome physical, physiological and pyschological chracteristics of patients with headache in Cochrane AL (ed): *Background to Migraine* London, Heineman, 1970; pp. 38-51.
5. Kudrow L: Physical and personality characteristics in cluster headache. *Headache* 1974; 13:197-201.
6. Kudrow L: The prevalence of migraine, peptic ulcer, coronary heart disease and hypertension in cluster headache. *Headache* 1976; 16:66-69.
7. Kudrow L, Sutkus BJ: MMPI patterns specificity in primary headache disorders. *Headache* 1979; 19:18-24.
8. Schele R, Ahlborg B, and Ekbom K: Physical characteristics and allergy history in young men with migraine and other headaches. *Headache* 1978; 18:80-86.
9. Ekbom K: Heart rate, blood pressure and electrocardiographic changes during provoked attacks of cluster headache. *Acta Neurol Scand* 1970; 46:215-224.
10. Ekbom K, Lindahl J: Effects of induced rise of blood pressure and pain on cluster headache. *Acta Neurol Scand* 1970; 46:586-600.
11. Steinhilber RM, Pearson JS, Rushton JG: Some psychological considerations of histaminic cephalgia. *Proc Staff Meet Mayo Clin* 1960; 35:691-699.

12. Rogado A, Harrison RH, Graham JR: Personality profiles in cluster headache, migraine and normal controls. Presented at the 10th International Congress of World Federation of Neurology, Sept 1973.
13. Friedman AP, Mikropoulous HE: Cluster headaches. *Neurology* 1958; 8:653-663.
14. Horton BT: Histaminic cephalgia (Horton's headache or syndrome). *Maryland Med J* 1961; 10:178-203.
15. Lance JW: Mechanism and management of headache ed 3. London, Butterworth, 1978.
16. Saper JR: Winters M, Van Meter MJ: Non-headache features in cluster headache patients. *Headache* 1981; 21:123-124.
17. Ekbom K, Greitz T: Carotid angiography and cluster headache. *Acta Radiol.* 1970; 10:177-186.
18. Lance JW, Anthony M: Migrainous neuralgia or cluster headaches? *J. Neurol Sci* 1971; 13:401.
19. Daniell HW: A study in the epidemiology of "crows feet." *Ann Intern. Med* 1971; 75:873-880.
20. Carney RG: Eye color in atopic dermatitis. *Arch Dermatol* 1962; 85:17-20.
21. Olesen J: Cluster headache associated with primary hyperlipidemia. *Acta Neurol Scand* 1977; 56:461-464.
22. Ekbom K: A clinical comparison of cluster headache and migraine. *Acta Neurol Scand* 1970; 4146 (suppl):1-48.
23. Ekbom K: Migraine in patients with cluster headache. *Headache* 1974; 14:69-72.
24. Horton BT: Histaminic cephalgia resulting in production of acute duodenal ulcer. *JAMA* 1943; 122:59.
25. Alford RI, Whitehous FR: Histaminic cephalgia and duodenal ulcer. *Amer Allerg* 1945; 3:200-203.
26. Lovshin LL: Clinical caprices of histaminic cephalgia. *Headache* 1961; 1: 7-10.
27. Ekbom KA: Ergotamine tartrate orally in Horton's histaminic cephalgia (also called Harris's ciliary neuralgia) *Acta Psychiat Scand* 1947; 46:106-113.
28. Ekbom K, Kugelberg E: Upper and lower cluster headache (Horton's syndrome). In Brain and Mind Problems. pp. 482-489 Il Pensiero Scientifico Publishers Ltd. Rome, 1978.
29. Ekbom K: Patterns of cluster headache with a note on the relations to angina pectoris and peptic ulcer. *Acta Neurol Scand* 1970; 46:225-237.
30. Graham JR: Proc. Conference on Cluster Headache. Proceedings of Headache Research Foundation, Faulkner Hospital, Massachusetts, 1968.
31. Graham JR: Discussion Bergen Migraine Symposium, June 1975.
32. Jacobson LB: Cluster headache: a rare cause of bradycardia. *Headache* 1969; 8:159-161.
33. Bruyn GW, Bootsma BK, and Klawans HL: Cluster headache and bradycardia. *Headache* 1976; 16:11-15.
34. Ekbom K: Heart rate, blood pressure and electrocardiographic changes during provoked attacks of cluster headache. *Acta Neurol Scand* 1970; 46:215-224.
35. Ekbom K: Nitroglycerin as a provocative agent in cluster headache. *Arch Neurol* 1968; 19:487-493.

36.   Rosenthal M: *Diseases of the Nervous System.* New York, William Wood, 1971, vol 2, pp. 254-256.
37.   Symonds CA: A particular variety of headache. *Brain* 1956; 79:217-232.

5
Peripheral Autonomic Abnormalities in Cluster Headache

N. VIJAYAN AND CRAIG WATSON

SYNOPSIS

Signs of disturbed autonomic function constitute a prominent feature of cluster headache. These include conjunctival injection, lacrimation, ptosis, miosis, nasal stuffiness and rhinorrhea. The differential role of parasympathetic and sympathetic pathways in the genesis of these signs and whether the location of lesion of these fibers is central or peripheral have been controversial. This review deals with the details of these clinical manifestations and presents evidence supporting that these "cluster accompaniments" are the result of peripheral sympathetic involvement, most likely in the pericarotid region.

INTRODUCTION

Evidences of peripheral autonomic dysfunction are often described in association with vascular headache syndromes like migraine[1] and pericarotid (Raeder's) syndrome[2]. These manifestations are a prominent feature in cluster headache and are often helpful in establishing a correct diagnosis. The exact pathogenesis of these signs is controversial. The clues these signs might provide in the delineation of the pathogenesis of cluster headache remain speculative.

Table 1. Peripheral Autonomic Signs in Cluster Headache.

Most Common	Conjunctival injection
	Lacrimation
	Nasal stuffiness
	Rhinorrhea
Less Common	Ptosis
	Miosis
Least Common	Mydriasis
	Facial hyperhidrosis
	Facial flushing
Probable	Cardiovascular changes
	Gastrointestinal

CLINICAL FEATURES

The most prominent feature of cluster headache, namely, the excruciating periorbital pain, is considered to be secondary to dilatation of the extracranial vasculature[3-5]. The role played by the autonomic nervous system in the pathogenesis of this vasodilatation is unknown at this time. Therefore, this topic is not discussed.

The associated manifestations of cluster headache are thought to be secondary to involvement of the autonomic nervous system, either centrally or peripherally. These are often designated as the "cluster accompaniments." These autonomic signs are summarized in Table 1.

These manifestations are discussed individually with regard to their incidence and relevant clinical features. Pathogenesis is discussed separately.

Conjunctival Injection and Lacrimation

These two symptoms occur simultaneously most often and therefore will be discussed together. These two manifestations are mentioned in what may possibly be considered as the earliest documentation of cluster headache in the literature by Romberg in 1840[6]. These occur usually along with the onset of pain and the severity of these symptoms seems to increase and peak along with the pain. These signs are almost always ipsilateral but Lance and Anthony have described it bilaterally in 5% of their patients[7]. Conjunctival vessels become dilated. The area around the limbus remains relatively clear. These changes subside along with the subsidence of pain but some injection remains for a variable period of time, usually minutes, after

Table 2. Conjunctival Injection and Lacrimation

Authors (year)	No. of patients	Frequency (%)
Symonds (1956)[8]	17	50
Kunkle and Anderson (1960)[9]	90	75
Ekbom (1970)[10]	105	87
Kudrow (1980)[11]	50	81
Manzoni et al (1981)[12]	76	85
Vijayan and Watson (1982)[13]	44	84

the pain has completely stopped. These are the most common accompaniments but are not invariably present as can be seen from the reports in the literature which are summarized in Table 2.

Nasal Symptoms

The two common nasal symptoms are ipsilateral stuffiness and rhinorrhea. The stuffiness may sometimes precede the actual onset of pain but most often starts along with the onset of pain. Some patients complain of the nose being unduly clear or dry so that they feel the air passing through the nose being colder on the involved side before the onset of the pain. It is sometimes also described as a "crawling" sensation in the nose. Nasal discharge usually increases later during the course of the pain and sometimes begins to subside. The discharge is clear and colorless. Drainage of tears into the nasal cavities at least partly contributes to the discharge. In all of our patients with rhinorrhea there was associated tearing. The frequency of nasal symptoms is shown in Table 3.

There appears to be a greater variability in the occurrence of nasal symptoms in the different series compared to conjunctival injection and lacrimation. It is possible that this is due to the fact that

Table 3. Nasal Symptoms in Cluster Headache

Authors (year)	No. of patients	Frequency (%)
Symonds (1956)[8]	17	30
Ekbom (1970)[10]	105	68
Kudrow (1980)[11]	50	72
Manzoni et al. (1981)[12]	76	33
Vijayan and Watson (1982)[13]	44	77

Table 4. Ptosis and Miosis in Cluster Headache

Authors (year)	No. of patients	Frequency (%)
Kunkle and Anderson (1960)[9]	90	15
Neiman and Hurwitz (1961)[15]	50	22
Ekbom (1970)[10]	105	18
Kudrow (1980)[11]	50	60
Manzoni et al (1981)[12]	76	53
Vijayan and Watson (1982)[13]	44	59

the nasal symptoms are often not as prominent as the eye symptoms and because they are less often enquired into specifically.

Ptosis and Miosis

Miosis as an accompaniment was first mentioned by Romberg in 1840[6]. Harris also described oculosympathetic paralysis but did not provide any figures regarding its frequency in his earlier descriptions[14]. Similarly Horton did not discuss miosis or ptosis in his original description in 1939[3]. The most detailed description of these manifestations was first provided by Kunkle and Anderson[9]. Table 4 provides a summary of subsequent reports.

Among these reports Kudrow[11] and Manzoni et al[12] mention only ptosis and not miosis. A dissociation between the ptosis and miosis has been recorded by Kunkle[9]. He found miosis alone in six patients and ptosis and miosis in eight patients. Both of these signs are often very mild and have to be specifically looked for. Otherwise it is easy for these manifestations to be missed. Another interesting observation is that these manifestations occur only during the cluster periods and may even disappear between each individual headaches. Often patients overlook these changes and have to be instructed to look for them during the headache. These may become evident only after the headaches have been occurring for a few few days. In some patients these changes outlast the cluster episodes and sometimes remain permanently.

Mydriasis, Facial Hyperhidrosis and Facial Flushing

Mydriasis during a cluster headache has been mentioned in individual case reports on rare occasions[9]. This is a very rare phenomenon and no detailed documentation regarding its frequency is known.

Table 5. Altered Facial Sweating in
Cluster Headache

Total no. reporting	13/44
Increased, bilateral	9
Increased, ipsilateral	2
Decreased, bilateral	1
Decreased, ipsilateral	1

Facial hyperhidrosis is occasionally reported by patients during the pain[15,17]. In our series of 44 patients, altered facial sweating was reported by 13 patients[13]. Mostly this information was obtained historically. Table 5 provides details of sweating changes in our patients.

As can be seen from this data, out of the 30% reporting an alteration of sweating, a majority had an increase bilaterally. It is unlikely that this is in any way specific. As it is bilateral, it most likely represents a response to the severe pain. Unilateral decreased or increased sweat response reported by the smaller number of patients is interesting. More detailed study of these changes may provide some clues regarding the nature of autonomic involvement in these patients. A recent study, using a method of measuring evaporation, found an increase of sweating along the ipsilateral medial forehead in eight out of 31 spontaneously occurring cluster headaches[18].

Facial "flushing" has been included as an associated manifestation of cluster headache in the description provided by the Ad Hoc Committee on the Classification of Headache[19]. Horton also mentioned this in his description[3]. Lance and Anthony described this in 20% of their patients[7]. Ekbom did not observe flushing in 45 spontaneous or induced attacks[10] and neither did Kudrow report this in 100 attacks of cluster headache[11]. In an editorial these two authors[10,11] suggested that the facial flushing is most likely secondary to application of pressure to the painful site rather than a spontaneous associated phenomenon[20]. None of our 44 patients reported facial flushing.

Cardiovascular Changes

Bradycardia has been described in patients during cluster headaches, mostly as isolated case reports[9,21-23]. The most detailed study of pulse and blood pressure changes was undertaken by Ekbom in 25 cluster patients in whom attacks were precipitated by nitroglycerin. He observed significant reduction in pulse rate and elevation of both systolic and diastolic blood pressure measurements. Both these changes correlated well with the severity of pain. He concluded that the bradycardia was most likely secondary to activation of the oculo-cardiac reflex mediated through the trigemino-vagal pathways. The elevation of blood pressure was thought to be secondary to activation of sympathetic response to pain[24]. Therefore, these changes are not considered to be due to direct autonomic disturbances as in the case of the other accompaniments.

Remission of intermittent claudication and angina pectoris have been reported during cluster headache attack[25,26]. The significance of these isolated case reports is not clear.

Gastrointestinal Changes

An increased incidence of peptic ulcer disease has been reported in patients with cluster headache[27-31]. The reported frequency has varied between 13% and 22%. The secretion rates have been found to sometimes approach that seen in Zollinger-Ellison syndrome[30] which is secondary to excessive production of gastrin. The significance of this again remains unknown but cannot be directly attributed to any specific neural influences. The marked stress of the attacks must play more of a role in the genesis of peptic ulcer disease than any other hormonal or neural mechanisms which might be operative.

PATHOGENESIS

The pathogenesis of these accompaniments has remained controversial. There are a number of unanswered questions still. Some of the recently published work may provide answers to a number of these questions.

It is fair to assume that most of the accompaniments described above are due to autonomic dysfunction. The first question to answer is whether this autonomic involvement is central or peripheral. Central involvement has been suggested to be the most likely answer in a recent discussion[32]. An increase in parasympathetic and decrease in sympathetic activity have been invoked at a central hypothalamic level to explain these accompaniments. No explanation has been offered for the well localized nature of these abnormalities. Most of the other authors support the idea that these accompaniments are due to peripheral autonomic involvement[9,15,33-35,13]. Ekbom and Grietz[33] found possible swelling of the internal carotid

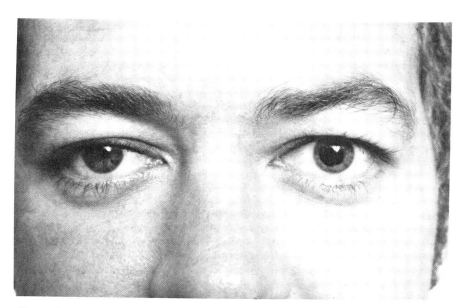

Figure 1.   Note the lack of response of the right pupil to hydroxyamphetamine 1% (Paredrine).

arterial wall on angiography during cluster headache in one patient. This observation resulted in the idea that the swollen vessel wall might cause compression of the pericarotid sympathetic plexus leading to these manifestations. Most of the other authors have come to this conclusion based solely on the clinical manifestations of ptosis and miosis. Lance[34] also suggested that there could be a decreased flow through the internal carotid in cluster patients based on the observation of the "cold spots" over the ipsilateral supraorbital region during cluster headache. These spots are very similar to what is observed in patients with internal carotid occlusion. This thesis has since then been corroborated by the Doppler studies of Kudrow[11] who concluded that "ipsilateral ophthalmic-supraorbital arterial flow may be diminished during interim and attack states of cluster headache."

More direct evidence has been presented by Vijayan and Watson[13] in support of the idea that the sympathetic fibers are involved peripherally and that the location of involvement is at a level beyond the bifurcation of the common carotid artery. Autonomic function was studied in seven cluster patients using well-established neuro-

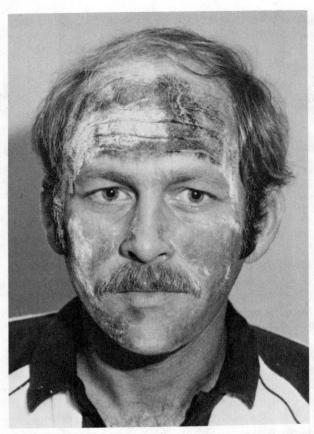

Figure 2. This illustrates the absent sweat response over the right supra-orbital region.

pharmacological and physiological tests[36]. Pupillary testing, using hydroxyamphetamine, revealed evidence of third neuronal lesion as indicated by the lack of response of the affected pupil (Fig. 1). It was also established that within the third neuron the location of the lesion could be further narrowed down to an area beyond the bifurcation of the common carotid. This was supported by the finding of a small area of anhidrosis over the ipsilateral forehead (Fig. 2). Therefore, one can conclude that the sympathetic fibers are damaged peripherally and that the location of this damage is between the bifurcation of the common carotid and the cavernous sinus. By inference, the most logical location will be in the petrous portion of

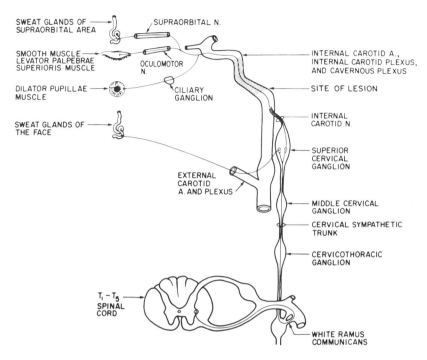

Figure 3.   Schematic diagram of the sympathetic pathways involved in cluster headaches. The shaded area represents the probable site of lesion.

the internal carotid where the pericarotid fibers could be easily compressed against the bony confines of the carotid canal (Fig. 3). This location also fits with the angiographic findings of Ekbom and Grietz[33] quoted earlier. Riley and Moyer have also reported in the past that the lesion responsible for miosis and ptosis in cluster headache is in the third neuronal pathway[37]. These findings, therefore, are very strong arguments against a central location for the autonomic dysfunction, at least as far as the cluster accompaniments are concerned.

Now that we have established that these manifestations are due to peripheral autonomic dysfunction, the next question is whether sympathetic hypofunction alone can explain these accompaniments or whether an associated parasympathetic involvement has to be considered. For purposes of this discussion, the cardiovascular changes described above will not be considered, as these have been found to be secondary to indirect effects of pain[24]. Peptic ulcer disease also will be excluded from this discussion because it is not a consistent phenomenon and its significance in relation to autonomic involvement is questionable.

Miosis and ptosis can be attributed to sympathetic deficit. Conjunctival injection and nasal stuffiness also can be attributed to sympathetic hypofunction. It is well known that sympathomimetic agents cause nasal and conjunctival vasoconstriction. A lesion of these fibers would therefore lead to conjunctival injection and nasal stuffiness. Guanethedine, which depletes norepinephrine from sympathetic terminals has been shown to cause conjunctival vasodilatation when applied locally[38]. Lacrimation and rhinorrhea cannot be attributed directly to sympathetic hypofunction. There is no doubt that the secretory functions of the lacrimal and nasal mucosal glands are controlled by parasympathetic fibers contained in the greater (superficial) petrosal nerve. The most direct evidence for this comes from the fact that cluster patients who continued to have their headaches following therapeutic resection of this nerve, did not have lacrimation and rhinorrhea as part of their headache. An alternative explanation is possible, though speculative, to explain these two features without invoking parasympathetic hyperactivity. Local irritation of the conjunctiva is the most common cause of tearing. Severe pain of the headache and the irritation due to marked conjunctival vasodilatation could be significant factors responsible for the excess tearing. Similarly, vasodilatation in the nose, along with the drainage of tears into the nose, could be sufficient cause for the rhinorrhea. This explanation is supported by our finding that 36 out of the 38 patients with tearing had conjunctival injection and that all patients with rhinorrhea reported tearing[13]. This explanation is still compatible with the loss of these two manifestations in cluster patients following greater (superficial) petrosal neurectomy because intact nerve supply to these glands is necessary to cause the excess secretion.

CONCLUSION

In summary, it can be stated that there is evidence of peripheral autonomic dysfunction in cluster headache. This dysfunction occurs at the third neuronal level and is most likely located in the pericarotid arterial sympathetic plexus in the region of the carotid canal. Miosis, ptosis, conjunctival injection and nasal stuffiness can be attributed directly to this sympathetic hypofunction. Lacrimation and rhinorrhea could be the indirect result of conjunctival and nasal vasodilatation. It is not necessary to attribute these symptoms to additional parasympathetic hyperactivity.

REFERENCES

1. Jacobson H: Unilateral sympathetic hypofunction in migraine. *Acta Neurol Scand* 1952; 27:67-83.
2. Vijayan N, Watson C: Pericarotid syndrome. *Headache* 1978; 18:244-254.
3. Horton BT, MacLean AR, Craig WM: A new syndrome of vascular headache: Results of treatment with histamine: Preliminary report. *Proc Staff Meet Mayo Clin* 1939; 14:257-260.
4. Kunkle EC, Pfeiffer JB Jr, Wilhoit WM Hamrick LW Jr: Recurrnet brief headache in cluster pattern. *Tr Am Neurol A* 1952; 77:240-243.
5. Lance JW, Anthony M: Thermographic studies in vascular headache. *Med J Aust* 1971; 1:240-243.
6. Romberg MH: A Manual of Nervous Diseases in Man, Sieveking EH (trans). London, Sydenham Society, 1840.
7. Lance JW, Anthony M: Migrainous neuralgia or cluster headache? *J. Neurol Sci* 1971; 13:401-414.
8. Symonds C: A particular variety of headache. *Brain* 1956; 79:217-232.
9. Kunkle EC, Anderson WB: Dual mechanisms of eye signs of headache in cluster pattern. *Tr Am Neurol A* 1960; 85:75-79.
10. Ekbom K: A clinical comparison of cluster headache and migraine. *Acta Neurol Scand* 1970; 46(suppl 41):1-48.
11. Kudrow L: *Cluster headache: Mechanisms and management.* New York, Oxford University Press, 1980.
12. Manzoni GC, Terzano MG, Moretti G, Cocchi M: Clinical observations in 76 cluster headache cases. *Eur Neurol* 1981; 20:80-94.
13. Vijayan N, Watson C: Evaluation of oculoephalic sympathetic function in vascular headache syndromes: Part 2—Oculocephalic sympathetic function in cluster headache. *Headache* 1982; 22:200-202.
14. Harris W: Neuritis and neuralgia. London, Oxford University Press, 1926.
15. Nieman EA, Hurwitz LJ: Ocular sympathetic palsy in periodic migrainous neuralgia. *J. Neurol Neurosurg Psychiatry* 1961; 24:369-373.
16. Duvoisian RC, Parker GW, Kenoyer WL: The cluster headache. *Arch Intern Med* 1961; 108:711-716.
17. Horton BJ: Histaminic cephalgia (Horton's headache or syndrome). *Maryland Med J* 1961; 10:178-203.
18. Sjaastad O, Russell D, Hestnes A, Marvik R: Cluster headache: The sweating pattern during spontaneous attacks. *Cephalagia* 1981; 1:233-244.
19. Ad Hoc Committee on classification of headache. *JAMA* 1962; 179:717-718.
20. Ekbom K, Kudrow L: Facial flush in cluster. *Headache* 1979; 19:47.
21. Dandy WE: Treatment of hemicrania by removal of the inferior cervical and first thoracic sympathetic ganglion. *Bull Johns Hop Hosp* 1931; 48:357-361.

22. Ekbom K, Kugelberg E: Upper and lower cluster headache (Horton's syndrome). In *Brain and Mind Problems* Rome Il Pensiero Sci. Publ. 1968; 482-489.
23. Jacobson LB: Cluster headache: a rare cause of bradycardia. *Headahce* 1969; 8:159-161.
24. Ekbom K: Heart rate, blood pressure and electrocardiographic changes during provoked attacks of cluster headache. *Acta Neurol Scand* 1970; 46:215-224.
25. Graham JR: Proceedings of conference on cluster headaches. Headache Research Foundation, Faulkner hospital, Boston, Massachusetts, 1968.
26. Ekbom K, Lindahl J: Remission of angina pectoris during periods of cluster headache. *Headache* 1971; 11:57-62.
27. Horton BJ: Histaminic cephalgia resulting in production of acute duodenal ulcer. *JAMA* 1943; 122:59.
28. Alford RI, Whitehouse FR: Histaminic cephalgia with duodenal ulcer. *Amer Allerg* 1945; 3:2000-2003.
29. Lovshin LL: Clinical caprices of histaminic cephalgia. *Headache* 1961; 1:7-10.
30. Graham JR: Cluster headache. *Headache* 1972; 11:175-185.
31. Kudrow L: Prevalence of migraine, peptic ulcer, coronary artery disease and hypertension in cluster headache. *Headache* 1976; 16:66-69.
32. Spierings ELH: The involvement of the autonomic nervous system in cluster headache. *Headache* 1980; 20:218-219.
33. Ekbom K, Grietz T: Carotid angiography in cluster headache. *Acta Radiol Diagn* 1970; 10:177-186.
34. Lance JW: Mechanism and Management of Headache, ed 3. London, Butterworth Scientific, 1980.
35. Sjaastad O: Pathogenesis of the cluster headache syndrome. *Res Clin Stud Headache* 1978; 6:53-64.
36. Watson C, Vijayan N: Evaluation of oculocephalic sympathetic function in vascular headache syndromes. Part 1—Methods of evaluation. Headache 1982; 22:192-199.
37. Riley FC, Moyer NJ: Oculosympathetic paresis associated with cluster headaches. *Amer J Opthal* 1971; 72:763-768.
38. Fanciullacci M: Iris adrenergic impairment in idiopathic headache. *Headache* 1979; 19:8-13.

6
Pathophysiologic Aspects of Cluster Headache

JOHN EDMEADS

CLUSTER HEADACHES AS VASCULAR HEADACHES

From the time of its delineation as a syndrome, there was little doubt in the minds of most clinicians that cluster headaches are vascular in origin. The persistent unilaterality of the headaches, their paroxysmal nature, their brevity, and their severity were reminiscent of migraine; and their precipitation by vasoactive substances such as histamine, alcohol and nitroglycerin, and occasional amelioration by ergotamine and methysergide reinforced this impression. There was some question of whether cluster headaches are intracranial vascular headaches, extracranial vascular headaches, or both. Some clinicians encountered local tenderness of the external carotid vessels during cluster headaches. Other workers[1] established that in some cases the pain of cluster headache could be relieved by raising intracranial (CSF) pressure, a maneuver which would affect only the intracranial circulation. Temple Fay[2] demonstrated that stimulation of the carotid artery bifurcation and of the origin of the internal carotid artery could produce pain in the same regions affected by cluster headache.

The presence of a neurogenic component in cluster headache was also recognized clinically from the first. The not uncommon occurrence of a partial Horner's syndrome, with sparing of facial sweating, suggested involvement of the sympathetic plexus investing the internal carotid artery; and the pupillary responses to cocaine and neo-synephrine indicated that the neural dysfunction is on the basis of

57

sympathetic palsy rather than parasympathetic hyperactivity. To complicate matters, however, the nasal discharge and blocking and the lacrimation which typically accompany cluster headache have been interpreted as suggesting parasympathetic hyperactivity (the autonomic aspects of cluster headache are covered in detail by Vijayan in this text.

Finally, there is considerable clinical evidence that there is more to cluster headaches than one carotid tree and the autonomic influences acting upon it. The increased incidence of peptic ulceration in cluster headache, the peculiar leonine facies seen in some patients with cluster, and the occasional occurrence of bradycardia, hypertension and EKG changes in spontaneous and induced attacks of cluster headache[3] all indicate that, like migraine, cluster headache has widespread systemic reverberations (see the chapter by Saper).

Clinical observations, therefore, suggest that cluster headaches emanate from the carotid system, likely the internal carotid; that autonomic influences are important; and that the syndrome is associated with generalized humoral and/or neurogenic changes which are capable of affecting other parts of the body.

THE HEMODYNAMICS OF CLUSTER HEADACHES

Angiography

Most workers have reported normal cerebral angiograms in patients with cluster headache. Nieman and Hurwitz[4] found no abnormality in ten patients with cluster headache, none of whom were studied during an attack. The single case of Sutherland and Eadie[5] was normal between attacks, as was the single case of Norris et al[6] ten minutes before an attack. Serratrice et al[7] reported normal carotid angiography in one patient during an attack of chronic cluster headache.

Ekbom and Greitz[8] demonstrated "ectasia" of all vessels in four of eighteen patients examined between attacks of cluster headache; the other fourteen were normal. In another patient angiograms were normal just prior to an attack. Fifteen minutes later, during the cluster headache, angiograms revealed localized narrowing of the lumen of the extradural part of the internal carotid artery just beyond its exit from the carotid canal, and dilatation of the ophthalmic artery. As the headache eased, repeat angiography showed extension of the narrowing proximally into the upper part of the carotid canal. The authors interpreted these changes as segmental mural edema of the artery.

It should be appreciated that the changes documented by Ekbom and Greitz, though definite, were nonetheless slight and it is difficult to see how they could have been of much hemodynamic significance. (Indeed, the occurrence of "cerebral ischemic" phenomena in cluster headache is exceptionally rare). However, edema of the arterial wall could have stimulated local pain receptors producing pain referred to the ipsilateral periorbital region (as intimated by the work of Temple Fay[2], see above) and could produce compression of the sympathetic periarterial plexus causing a partial Horner's syndrome. It is essential of course to remember that this is a single case.

Cerebral Blood Flow Studies

The first measurement of regional cerebral blood flow (rCBF) during an attack of cluster headache was done only six years ago by Norris et al[6] using an intracarotid ^{133}Xe technique; they found rCBF increased throughout the single hemisphere measured, which was the hemisphere ipsilateral to the headache. Sakai and Meyer,[9] using an inhalation ^{133}Xe technique (which records rCBF simultaneously in both hemispheres and which, using appropriate computations, can estimate blood flow in the extracerebral compartment) studied nine patients, seven during cluster headaches. They found rCBF increased, more so contralateral to the headache, with the increase subsiding promptly as the pain subsided. (This could represent merely activation of the contralateral cortex by pain perception). Sakai and Meyer also noted an increase in extracerebral blood flow of greater magnitude than the increases encountered in migraine, higher on the side of the head pain; they inferred that the pain of cluster headache might originate from hyperemia of the extracerebral vessels.

However, other workers have not been able to demonstrate an invariable increase of rCBF during cluster headache. Henry, Vernheit et al,[10] using an intracarotid ^{133}Xe technique, studied three patients during cluster headaches with normal results. Nelson, du Boulay et al[11] employed an intravaenous ^{133}Xe clearance technique to study twenty-six patients with cluster headache (thirteen during spontaneous or induced headaches, the others between headaches) and found such a mixture of increased rCBFs, decreased rCBFs, and normal rCBFs that they could discern no pattern.

Yamamoto and Meyer[12] studied the effects on rCBF in cluster headache patients of substances capable of selectively blocking or stimulating the alpha and beta adrenergic receptors of the cerebral blood vessels. They found that those substances which affected the adrenoceptors directly (i.e., "peripherally acting adrenergics") exerted more effect on the vessels of the side of the most recent headache, while centrally acting agents exerted more effect on the non-headache side. They felt that there was an asymmetric adrenoceptor disorder in migraine and cluster headache, probably related to sympathetic denervation hypersensitivity. It is not clear whether this possible sympathetic denervation is a cause or an effect of the recurrent headaches.

In summary, the high technology of the cerebral blood flow laboratory, while it has provided some data suggesting that there may at times be dysfunction of the cranial vasculature in cluster headache, has on the whole yielded disappointingly few insights into the vascular pathophysiology of cluster headache.

Doppler Studies

Kudrow[13] measured the velocity of blood flow through the supraorbital artery, on both sides of the head, between and during attacks of cluster headaches. These arteries are the terminal cutaneous branches of the *internal* carotid artery. A change in the velocity of flow in these arteries could be due to obstructive disease in the trunk of the internal carotid artery, primary changes in the supraorbital artery (e.g., vasoconstriction) or increased pressure in those branches of the external carotid artery which anastomose with the supraorbital arteries, increasing the "resistance to outflow" of the supraorbital arteries. In most of his patients Kudrow found decreased flow velocity on the headache side between attacks; a further decrease on the side of the headache during the headache; increase in flow velocity 10 to 15 minutes after the administration of ergotamine; and reduction towards baseline after an hour. These results have been interpreted by some as suggesting "carotid trunk" constriction, but (as noted above) could conceivably be produced by small vessel changes or even external carotid changes.

Thermography

This technique is based on the premise that skin temperature is a product of cutaneous blood flow; the higher the flow the higher the temperature, the lower the flow the lower the temperature.

Friedman et al[14] showed that approximately 85% of patients with cluster headache have "cold spots" in the skin of the forehead ipsilateral to the pain. In some cases these cold spots are maximal in that part of the skin supplied by the ophthalmic (i.e. internal carotid) artery; in others they are prominent on the watershed between this area and the area supplied by the external carotid artery. These cold spots are approximately one degree centigrade cooler than the surrounding skin; they are approximately 0.5 centimeters in diameter; they are usually multiple; biopsy of skin containing a cold spot is unremarkable; angiograms in patients with cold spots are normal (making it extremely unlikely that they are due to carotid narrowing). These cold spots persist between headaches and are not more prominent during headaches.

These cold spots likely represent reduced cutaneous blood flow, and may be produced either by constriction of the supraorbital and supratrochlear arteries or their branches, or by arteriovenous shunting within the skin.

In his thermographic studies Lance[15] has found that the temperature of the skin supplied by the internal carotid artery is reduced compared to its (external carotid supplied) surroundings at the start of the attack, and that later in the attack there is an increase of temperature in these surroundings. Kudrow's thermographic studies[13] have confirmed a decrease in temperature in untreated and unsuccessfully treated patients during an attack, with subsequent increase in skin temperature in successfully treated patients.

Corneal Indentation Pulse Patterns

In this application of dynamic tonometry the corneal indentation pulse (CIP) amplitude reflects the volume of blood pumped into the eye with each systole. The technique, however, does not allow any inference about total blood flow through the eye, since this depends on the small vessels. For example, if vasoconstriction occurred in the distal portion of the ocular vessels, dilatation and increased pulsation of the proximal portions might occur in an attempt to overcome the increased peripheral resistance. Horven et al[16] have demonstrated that in cluster headache patients there is a tendency, between attacks, for the CIP to be increased on the "headache side"; during headaches it increases further. In migraine, in contrast, there is a minor decrease of CIP between attacks and a further decrease during attacks.

Summary of Hemodynamic Changes

In a single case, angiography has demonstrated what might be a minor degree of mural edema during the headache of a segment of the internal carotid artery as it traverses the base of the skull. The lumenal narrowing so formed is clearly insufficient to produce any hemodynamic effect. Recordings of cerebral blood flow give no consistent results. Doppler studies and cutaneous thermography suggest that even between attacks there may be changes in flow through the cutaneous branches of the internal carotid artery on the side of the headache. Corneal indentation pulse pattern recordings suggest that there is also a change, difficult to interpret, in the intrinsic circulation of the eye on the headache side. Presumably all these circulatory changes are on the basis of alterations in the smaller blood vessels. Many of the techniques used yield results that are subject to more than one interpretation and it is not possible at this time to make a plausible synthesis of this heterogenous data.

HUMORAL FACTORS IN THE PRODUCTION OF CLUSTER HEADACHES

Given that there are hemodynamic changes in cluster headache, these may be produced by neurogenic or humoral factors. The neurogenic aspects of cluster headaches are dealt with by Dr. Vijayan (this text). Some of the humoral factors investigated in cluster headache follow.

Histamine

Horton,[17] noting the precipitation of attacks of cluster headache in susceptible individuals by histamine, and the apparent successful treatment of some cases by a histamine desensitizaion procedure, implicated histamine in the etiology of this condition. This is a somewhat tenuous argument since substances other than histamine may also trigger cluster headaches, and since other workers have at times found it difficult to reproduce Horton's success with histamine desensitization.

Sjaastad and Sjaastad[18] found increased amounts of histamine in the urine of about a third of their patients with cluster headaches on the days of their attacks. They administered C14-labelled histamine to their subjects and noted no discernible abnormality of histamine metabolism. The possibility was considered that increased urine histamine might be a result rather than a cause of the attacks. Anthony and Lance[19] found that whole blood histamine levels were 20% higher in patients with cluster headache than they were in migraine patients and in control subjects (blood histamine levels were the same in the latter two groups). Medina, Diamond and Fareed[20] documented increased histamine levels in platelet rich plasma (prp) prepared from blood from the general venous circulation (antecubital vein). As well, there was a "nonstatistically significant but interesting" decrease in prp histamine in blood from the jugular vein ipsilateral to the headache; the authors comment that one of the characteristics of the blood vessels on the side of the pain may be an avidity for histamine.

Prusinski and Liberski[21] performed skin biopsies of the painful areas of thirteen cluster headache patients, comparing them with nine controls, and counted the mast cells (which contain histamine). There was a significant increase in mast cells in the skin on the side of the cluster headaches. This was a light microscopy study and there was no comment re degranulation of the mast cells. Appenzeller et al,[22] in an ultrastructural study, found increased numbers of mastocytes in the painful areas, but they were not degranulated (this may be due to biopsies being taken between rather than during attacks). The meaning of these skin studies is not clear. Mast cells are present in the intracranial vessles, but we do not know whether the cutaneous mastocytosis mirrors a similar change in the blood vessels.

Histamine does affect blood vessels of the external carotid tree in vitro, at least in the patients with primary chronic cluster headaches whose superficial temporal artery sections were studied by Hardebo et al.[23] The vasodilatation produced by histamine seemed to be mediated via the H2 receptors. It is difficult to apply this in vitro work to the clinical setting, of course, because the in vitro technique involves stimulation of both lumenal and extralumenal sites by the histamine.

Possibly the definitive test of the role of histamine in cluster headache is the response of patients with this condition to a combination of H1 and H2 blockers. Anthony, Lord and Lance[24] found in a controlled study that combinations of chlorpheniramine and cimetidine had no effect on cluster headache. Even this may not permit final rejection of histamine as an important factor in the genesis of cluster headache, The authors point out that histamine may be produced within the cell by the decarboxylation of histidine. This intracellular histamine would not be susceptible to histamine receptor blockade. They suggest that interference with the local production of histamine might be a more effective treatment, and cite the ability of corticosteroids to block the enzyme histidine decarboxylase.

Despite the extensive work done on histamine, therefore, there is still no conclusive evidence of its significance in the pathogenesis of cluster headache. There is a general impression, however, that histamine is somehow involved.

Serotonin

This amine, while considered important in migraine, seems to play no major role in cluster headache. Anthony and Lance[19] found no change in the serotonin levels of their patients. Medina, Diamond and Fareed[20] did find, however, increased platelet serotonin in the general venous circulation of their patients with cluster headaches, and a decreased number of platelets in the jugular venous blood ipsilateral to the headache.

Prostaglandins

These seem not to be important in cluster headache. Bennett et al[25] did not note any increase in prostaglandin levels during attacks of cluster headache, and Peatfield et al[26] were unable to trigger cluster headaches in susceptible individuals by infusing prostacyclin.

Acetylcholine

The lacrimation, sweating and conjunctival suffusion that characterize cluster headaches suggested to Kunkle[27] the involvement of acetylcholine. He found "acetylcholinelike activity" in the CSF of five of eight cluster headache patients, none of twenty-two patients with other types of headaches, and none of thirty-seven controls. The meaning of these findings is not clear.

Endogenous Opioids

Anselmi et al[28] assayed the levels of encephalins in the CSF of patients with vascular headaches and in controls. In the five cluster headache patients studied, encephalins were undetectable, even in the intervals between headaches. In migraine CSF encephalins were slightly low between headaches, and lower but still detectable during headaches. It is not known whether the extremely low encephalin levels in cluster headache patients is due to decreased production or increased consumption.

Hormones

The strong male predisposition to cluster headache suggested to a number of workers that hormonal factors might be important in pathogenesis. *Testosterone* levels are either normal or very slightly diminished,[29] but it must be recalled that testosterone secretion may be depressed nonspecifically by chronic illness and by narcotic analgesics. There is no change in the levels of *TSH, RSH, GH, cortisol* or *prolactin*,[30] though Polleri et al[31] noted that in cluster headache patients the pattern of prolactin secretion may be abnormal, with loss of the usual sinusoidal rhythm. In terms of any possible relationship between cluster headache and *female sex hormones*, Ekbom and Waldenlind[32] have noted no relationship between cluster headache and menstruation, fewer cluster headaches during pregnancy, and fewer pregnancies in females with cluster headaches (though this last observation may be explained on the basis of Goldblatt's second phenomenon—"I have a headache. Not tonight.")[33]

AN EVALUATION OF HEMODYNAMIC AND HUMORAL DATA

Research into the pathogenesis of cluster headache seems characterized by much activity and by largely negative, marginal or irreproduceable results. There is not enough consistent data to present a convincing hypothesis.

Medina, Diamond and Fareed[20] have sketched an outline of a possible scenario in which a malfunctioning hypothalamic oscillator periodically unleashes a biochemical and/or neurogenic disturbance which acts upon a carotid system that is in an altered and therefore susceptible state, producing the intense vascular headaches which we term cluster headaches. The evidence for this is incomplete, but it is a plausible suggestion which indicates further investigation.

REFERENCES

1. Thomas WA, Butler S: Treatment of migraine by intravenous histamine. *Am J Med* 1946; 1:39-44.
2. Fay T: Atypical facial neuralgia, a syndrome of vascular pain. *Ann Otol Rhinol Laryngol* 1932; 41:1030-1062.

3. Ekbom K: Heart rate, blood pressure and electrocardiographic changes during provoked attacks of cluster headache. *Acta Neurol Scand* 1970; 46:214-224.
4. Nieman EA, Hurwitz LJ: Ocular sympathetic palsy in periodic migrainous neuralgia. *J Neurol Neurosurg Psychiat* 1961; 24:369-373.
5. Sutherland JM, Eadie MJ: Cluster headache. *Res Clin Stud Headache* 1972; 3:92-125.
6. Norris JW, Hachinski VC, Cooper PW: Cerebral blood flow changes in cluster headache. *Acta Neurol Scand* 1976; 54:371-374.
7. Serratrice G, Rascol A, Gastant JL, Layani M: Algies vasculaires de la face in Migraines et Céphalées. Sandoz Ediction 1972, p. 15.
8. Ekbom K, Greitz T: Carotid angiography in cluster headache. *Acta Radiol Diagn* 1970; 10:177-186.
9. Sakai F, Meyer JS: Regional cerebral hemodynamics during migraine and cluster headaches measured by the ^{133}Xe inhalation method. *Headache* 1978; 18:122-132.
10. Henry PY, Vernheit J, Orgogozo JM, Caille JM: Cerebral blood flow in migraine and cluster headache. *Res Clin Stud Headache* 1978; 6:81-88.
11. Nelson RF, du Boulay GH, Marshall J, Ross Russell RW, Symon L, Zilkha E: Cerebral blood flow studies in patients with cluster headache. *Headache* 1980; 20:184-189.
12. Yamamoto M, Meyer JS: Hemicranial disorder of vasomotor adrenoceptors in migraine and cluster headache. *Headache* 1980; 20:321-335.
13. Kudrow, L: Thermographic and doppler flow asymmetry in cluster headache. *Headache* 1979; 19:204-208.
14. Friedman AP, Wood EH, Rowan AJ et al: Observations on vascular headache of the migraine type, in *Background to Migraine, Fifth Migraine Symposium 1971.* Cummings JN (ed): London, William Heinemann Medical Books Ltd., 1973, p. 1-6.
15. Lance JW: Mechanism and Management of Headache, ed 3. London, Butterworth Scientific, 1978, p. 220.
16. Horven I, Nornes H, Sjaastad O: Different corneal indentation pulse patterns in cluster headache and migraine. *Neurology* 1972; 22:92-98.
17. Horton BT, MacLean AR, Craig WM: A new syndrome of vascular headache: result of treatment with histamine: Preliminary report. *Proc Staff Meet Mayo Clin* 1939; 14:257-260.
18. Sjaastad O, Sjaastad OV: Urinary histamine excretion in migraine and cluster headache. *J Neurol* 1977; 216:91-104.
19. Anthony M, Lance JW: Histamine and serotonin in cluster headache. *Arch Neurol* 1971; 25:225-231.
20. Medina JL, Diamond S, Fareed J: The nature of cluster headache. *Headache* 1979; 19:309-322.
21. Prusinski A, Liberski PO: Is the cluster headache a local mastocytic diathesis? *Headache* 1979; 19:102.
22. Appenzeller O, Becker W, Ragan A: Cluster headache: ultrastructural aspects. *Neurology* 1978; 28:371.
23. Hardebo JE, Krabbe AA, Gjerris F: Enhanced dilatory response to histamine in large extracranial vessels in chronic cluster headache. *Headache* 1980; 20:316-320.
24. Anthony M, Lord G, Lance JW: Controlled trials of cimetidine in migraine and cluster headache. *Headache* 1978; 18:261-264.

25. Bennett A, Magnaes B, Sandler M, Sjaastad O: Prostaglandins and headache in *Background to Migraine. Sixth Migraine Symposium.* London, Sept 26-27, 1974.
26. Peatfield RC, Gawel MJ, Clifford Rose F: The effect of infused prostacyclin in migraine and cluster headache. *Headache* 1981; 21:190-195.
27. Kunkle EC: Acetylcholine in the mechanisms of headaches of the migraine type. *Arch Neurol Psychiat* 1959; 81:135-140.
28. Anselmi B, Baldi E, Casacci F, Salmon S: Endogenous opioids in cerebrospinal fluid and blood in idiopathic headache sufferers. *Headache* 1980; 20:294-299.
29. Nelson RF: Testosterone levels in cluster and non-cluster migrainous headache patients. *Headache* 1978; 18:265-267.
30. Kudrow L: *Cluster Headache: Mechanisms and Management.* New York Oxford University Press, 1980.
31. Polleri A, Nappi G, Savoldi F: Prolactin secretion. *Headache* 1980; 20: 114-115.
32. Ekbom K, Waldenlind E: Cluster headache in women: Evidence of hypofertility (?). Headaches in relation to menstruation and pregnancy. *Cephalalgia* 1981; 1:167-174.
33. Goldblatt D: Of love, sleep and headache. *Sem in Neurol* 1981; 2:ii.

7
Cycles in Cluster Headache

JAMES D. DEXTER

The world in which we practice medicine is filled with cyclical phenomenon, the day (earth), the month (moon), the year (sun), all of
which we are quite adapted to and assume we understand; however,
some of the most difficult phenomena to understand in relationship
to headache are the cyclical phenomena which are associated with
headache. We can remind ourselves of two particularly frustrating
and pathophysiologically obscure forms of headache: menstrual
migraine and cluster headache. Both of these are the most firm examples of pathological cycles which remain obscure.

There are two types of cycles involved in the process of cluster
headache which by their characteristics appear to be quite different,
the annual occurrence of a cluster which may vary from three
months to several years, and the daily cycles or individual attack
cycles ranging from every several days to seven to ten per day. The
longer of the two cyclical phenomena is at this point quite obscure.
There are similar cycles which occur in gastrointestinal disease such
as peptic ulcers, however, there is no solid relationship between these
two diseases. Their predilection for spring and fall shows at least a
statistical cycle in both. The only statement that has validity is that
they may be related to biological adaptive processes and this argument is very weak, coming only from clinical impressions.

The individual attack cycle probably will be illucidated sooner
because of our growing understanding of circadian and sleep cycles.

Over the past three decades there has been a growing understanding of these cyclical changes; however, they have been a legitimate scientific pursuit for the last half century. They have become the basis of clinical pathology, i.e., so many of the measurable body constituents, particularly enzymes, have a daily variation that the standard clinical pathological specimen is collected in the first hour after awakening. In no area of biochemical physiology is this more striking than the pituitary hormones and rapid eye movement sleep, which have been extensively studied and may play a major contributing role in the patient with cluster headache.

These hormones have several types of patterns[1]: (1) Daily, nycterohemeral or circadian, (2) brief or episodic release, and (3) very slow or infradian. The pattern of the cluster headache is at such a varying frequency that it is impossible to theoretically incriminate any single hormone; however, those hormones which appear to have both nycterohemeral and episodic components may be the major offenders. Growth hormone has one such pattern which appears; it contains a primary peak shortly after sleep onset and several smaller peaks during the waking hours, and fits the pattern of cluster headache most closely. Prolactin appears to have a rapid release immediately following the onset of sleep. It appears to have more than an on/off response to sleep (high levels during sleep and in as much as this hormone may be related to the lower levels during the daytime hours). Thyrotropin may have several peaks during the day, however, there is a peak prior to the onset of sleep and a smooth disappearance during sleep which would not match the nocturnal pattern of cluster.

Cortisol has a somewhat smoother pattern and does appear to be unaffected by the REM cycles of sleep but does peak just prior to awaking, whereas testostereone and leutinizing hormone probably are more sporadic than the others and would be excellent candidates for effectors of the cluster cycles.

The naturally occurring physiological rhythms of the sleep/wake cycle probably serve as the most reasonable candidate for the origin of the cyclical pathology in the syndrome of cluster headache. The finding that nocturnal arousals with cluster headache attacks are related to the rapid eye movement (REM) stage of sleep[2] was the first documentation of an intrinsic rhythm related to cluster and allowed the central nervous system to be incriminated in the syndrome of cluster headache.

This REM/cluster relationship helps to explain the periodicity of nocturnal arousals; however, until Othmer et al[3] reported the observations that suggested the existence of REM like activity occurring in cycles during the day the physiological substrate of diurnal attacks of cluster remained obscure. There are no studies which relate daytime REM to the occurrence of cluster at this time; however, if those studies emerge and do show a relationship, then an understanding of the REM/non-REM cycle may be the key to the understanding of the syndrome of cluster headache.

The relationship of the autonomic features of cluster has recently been clarified by the investigations leading to the description of the central or internal autonomic nervous system, which has allowed us to better understand these sleep/autonomic nervous system relationships.

Until recently the investigator attempting to investigate the mechanisms of migraine was forced to assume that it was either the humoral triggering or cervical autonomic control. The recent investigations into the central autonomic system and the potential control of the small arteriolar tone has given rise to a new and broader view of the mechanism of migraine.[4]

The central adrenergic system, very well demonstrated by Swanson and Hartman,[5] which has its origin both in the diffuse pontine and medullary regions and in a well localized area, locus ceruleus. From these areas this system projects anteriorly to terminate both synaptically and as free boutons. The portion which has its origin in the locus coeruleus has been most investigated because of the precise localization and has been found by Raichle et al[6] to be analogous to the peripheral sympathetic system in its ability to effect both cerebral blood flow and vascular permeability.

With these observations it is now obvious that those humoral changes which have consumed the effort of so many excellent investigators in the past may in fact be descriptors of the peripheral effects of ongoing central activity. While there may be significant peripheral mechanisms, they may only reflect those secondary changes or responses to primary central nervous system changes which Lance[7] has postulated. Since this system is closely associated both anatomically and biochemically with the mechanisms of the sleep/wake cycle, well summarized by Jouvet,[8] it relates to the only physiological definable state which is associated with the onset of migraine, the arousal with headache in Rapid Eye Movement phase of sleep.

While the cyclical variation of the cluster headache syndromes are still obscure, there are many cyclical relationships which may be allowing us to gain a better understanding of the possible pathophysiology of cluster headache.

REFERENCES

1. Parker DC, et al: Endocrine rhythms across sleep-wake cycles in normal young men under basal state conditions, in Orem J and Barnes CD (eds): *Physiology in Sleep.* New York, Academic Press, 1980, pp. 145-179.
2. Dexter JD: The relationship between stage III & IV & REM sleep and arousals with migraine. *Headache* 1979; 19:364-369.
3. Othemer E, Hayden MP, and Segelbaum R: Encephalic cycles during sleep and wakefulness in humans: A 24-hour pattern. *Science* 1969; 164:447.
4. Raichle ME, Hartman BK, Eichling JO and Shrrpe LG. Central nonadrenergic regulation of cerebral blood flow and vascular permeability. *Proc Natn Acad Sci USA* 1975; 72:3626.
5. Swanson LW and Hartman BK. The central adrenergic system. An immunofluorscence study study of the location of cell bodies and their efferent connections in the rat utilizing dopamine-B-hydroxylase as a marker. *J Comp Neurol* 1975; 163:467-506.
7. Lance J: Mechanisms and management of headache. In *Mechanism and Management of Headache,* ed 4. 162. London, Butterworth Scientific, 1982, p 162
8. Jouvet M: Biogenic amines and the states of sleep. *Science* 1969; 163:32.

8
The Psychological and Behavioral Aspects of the Cluster Headache Patient

ARNOLD P. FRIEDMAN

Paroxysmal attacks of cluster headache have been well documented in the literature for over a hundred years under a variety of clinical entities, eponyms, and synonyms. Cluster headache is the only primary headache disorder in which affected males outnumber females. Most authors agree that neurological and physical examinations yield no abnormal findings with the possible exception of an ipsilateral Horner's syndrome. If abnormal signs are present they are probably due to some unrelated condition.

Headaches of psychological origin may produce symptoms in two different ways: indirectly, as symbolic attempts to solve problems, or directly, as alterations of specific physiological functions. These alterations are very often the physiologic expression of an existing emotional feeling or tension state.

Reports in the literature are not in full agreement as to the psychological background and personality patterns of these patients, nor is it possible to verify the exact role psychological factors play in their headache problem or if the primary etiology is psychogenic. Wolff regards the disease as closely related to true migraine and one of the many varieties of painful vascular disorders of the head. He emphasized that these headaches resemble migraine and are linked to one another in that they are all related to the patient's emotional conflicts and life's stresses. He presents detailed case reports correlating cessation of each cluster of pain with the opportunity for the

the patient to express resentments and conflicts to a sympathetic reassuring physician.

In 1958[1] my colleague, Doctor Mikropoulos, and I reported a detailed study of fifty patients with cluster headache and emphasized the importance of psychological factors. Although it was not possible in many of these patients to verify that the primary etiology was psychogenic, the importance of psychological factors in their headache problems could not be minimized.

The personality pattern most often observed was that of an adult who was ambitious, efficient, and overconscientious, strove toward perfection, and had a strong tendency toward compulsive behavior; in other words, a constitutional predisposition to sustained emotional states. They often had positions of responsibility, but were insecure and often had a lack of self-confidence in their ability. The most frequent conflicts observed were of a hostile and aggressive nature. A similar personality type is observed in patients who have classical migraine, hypertension, ulcers, or no illness. It was unusual to find that the initial painful attack occurred with a known disturbing emotional experience.

It was particularly interesting that many of these patients could not recognize that they were under greater stress, more emotionally upset or fatigued prior to an attack than in the preceding months or years. Furthermore, during their attacks they continued to work, in spite of pain, loss of sleep, and increased stress, which does not usually change the duration of each bout of cluster headache. They occur and continue whether the patient is at work or on vacation, on land, ocean, or desert, in warm or cold weather.

It is still undecided whether the resultant tension which develops from personality reactions to life can explain these attacks. However, it was our belief that they are closely related.

Charles Kunkle et al, in 1952,[2] thought that the bouts with pain of 30 patients followed their accompanied increased tension and conflict, and that there was chronic tension in about 50% of the patients. But of these only a few had a compulsive and driving temperament.

Graham[3] described his patients as "mice living inside lions." He drew attention to the connections between cluster headache and persons of a special constitutional type who were "go-getters" with aggressive behavior, masking feelings of dependency and inadequacy. They had enlarged facial bones producing a lionlike expression (Leontiasis Ossea) with ruddy complexion, thick facial skin (which he termed orange peel), visibly dilated blood vessels (particularly across the bridge of the nose), deeply furrowed forehead, a broad chin and skull and often they had relatively high hematocrit values. He also noted a high correspondence between cluster headache and a tall, trim, rugged body type.

His profile of the cluster headache male is a timid individual with strong hysterical streaks and increased dependency needs.

Among the patients myself and others have observed, such physical characteristics are not represented to any unusual extent. Other studies based on larger samples with more extensive personality probes puts this assessment in question.

Studies by Kudrow and his associates[4] did not confirm some of Graham's observations and added some other evidence to physical aspects of this problem. He found that migraine and cluster groups scored similarly on all scales of the MMPI; contrary to previous reports, there was no evidence of conversion configuration. Along with abnormally high proportions of hazel-eyed persons, there was an abnormally low proportion of blue-eyed persons. He suggested that cluster patients might also have in common some defect in the regulation of melanin, a pigment associated with eye and skin color. It is very questionable if this defect plays a role in causing headaches; it is possibly merely an additional symptom of some chemical disorder. He studied forty-one patients with cluster headache using the MMPI and found no significant differences from controls.

On the other hand, Lesse in 1963 thought that all fifty-three of his patients were intelligent, capable, aggressive, domineering, conscientious, and perfectionistic. All but three had moderate to severe depression. In all of his patients of both sexes he said that emotional stress preceded by many months the initial paroxysm of pain and that over twenty-five percent of his patients were in an emotional crisis at the time of onset of the syndrome. Moreover, there was a painfree period of one or more months with marked emotional pressure build-up before the symptoms recurred. Earlier he had studied seven patients in remission by giving intravenous drugs which would place the patient under emotional stress: mescaline to one, lysergic acid to two, and amphetamines to four. In five of these seven, a paroxysmal pain appeared as they showed marked anxiety.

Two forms of social behavior indirectly related to personality have been noted. Male cluster sufferers tend to smoke substantially more and drink more coffee and alcoholic beverage than men of ordinary good health. However, they usually abstain from alcohol during cluster episodes as even a small quantity is well-known to precipitate another attack. In this connection mention must also be made of the tendency to develop ulcers in cluster headache patients.

It must be emphasized that these statements are observations and have never been fully documented under carefully controlled studies of the general population or geographic areas.

Symonds[5] vigorously opposed the factor of stress. He remarked that no evidence could be attained for the assumption that psychological factors were operative. Out of seventeen of his patients, only two had obsessional tendencies with episodes of anxiety, but the bouts did not coincide with or follow periods of psychological tension.

Furthermore, out of forty-seven patients examined by Neiman and Hurwitz in 1961,[6] only seven regarded worry, overwork, or stress as provocative factors in their pain; Schiller in 1960[7] found only eight of his fifty-two patients to be suffering from anxiety or to have compulsive, phobic characteristics.

In 1960[8] Steinhilber et al concluded that their fifty patients with histaminic cephalagia showed a profile with a marked similarity to that of patients diagnosed as having conversion hysteria.

Marin et al in 1967 and 1972, and Rogado et al in 1973[9] gave the Minnesota Multiphasic Personality Inventory to selected outpatients who had cluster headache. Both headache groups reported more psychopathology than the control groups and the profiles of both migraine and cluster patients indicated the presence of obsessive, compulsive traits. Elevations of the hysteria scale were consistent with the dissociative behavior often observed in these headache patients. Both headache groups scored higher on the hypochondriasis and hysteria scale with moderate scores on depression. The headache groups did not differ significantly from the control groups on a scale indicating uncertainty in sex identification.

Other studies imprudently hold that special personality traits, other than anxiety, predispose to cluster headache. There is no doubt that anxious, obsessional, intelligent, and persistent patients are often found to have cluster headache, migraine, etc. Frazier has emphasized emotional disturbances, particularly anxiety and depression, as being related to the onset of the attacks. Until proven otherwise, this has to be regarded as an affective selection. However, emotional disturbances, emotional stress, anxiety, depression, and biochemical changes which are associated with affective illnesses may relate to the production of the attacks. To this extent there is likely a link between having an anxious personality and being somewhat liable to suffer headaches such as cluster headache or migraine. Whether this is their basic personality or their reaction to the stresses of a chronic painful disturbance has still not been proven.

Other types of headaches, which were not episodic or periodic, have been classified under cluster. This includes chronic cluster–primary chronic headache, because these patients do not have any remissions while those whose headaches became chronic have had specific episodic patterns which have been characterized as the secondary chronic type. According to Ekbom and Olivarus[10] and others, chronic cluster headache is distinguished from the episodic type by the absence of remission periods for at least one year. Also, attempts have been made to classify cluster migraine, an atypical variant of migraine having components of both disorders.

Chronic paroxysmal hemicrania, first described by Sjaastad and Dale in 1974,[11] has been included in this group differing from the chronic cluster in that all known cases are women, the attacks are more frequent, shorter in duration, and rarely occur during sleep hours. Recently Russell and Mathew[12] have added further cases to the total. It has been reported that both these types of cluster are dramatically responsive to aspirin and Indomethacin.

Chronic paroxysmal hemicrania has been reported by Medina and Diamond[13] as a cluster headache variant with brief, high daily frequency (15 or more attacks per day) which can be triggered by movement and respond to Indomethacin.

The occurrence of cluster headache with vertigo was first described by Gilbert in 1965[14]. Headache and vertigo attacks may share the same mechanism, recurrent paroxysmal multi-focal vasodilatation, but again all of these variants have some differences from the original classic periodic type. There is little evidence to support the idea that the occurrence of the headaches in these groups is psychological or that the sufferers have a specific personality or psychological profile.

Ekbom's delineation of a chronic syndrome is often claimed as the original description, but in fact Symonds paper[5] in 1956 on a particular type of headache clearly described a patient with chronic syndrome. McArdle in 1959 described similar features at the British Migraine Symposium and discussed the role of trigeminal destructive procedures in his treatment.

I have seen a number of these patients during the last forty years. However, the limits of value in differentiating these types really depends upon their treatment response and I found that most of these patients reacted very much like the periodic typical cluster patient.

If anything is clear from this discussion of cluster headache, it is that despite multiple studies, theories, and observations, there remains much controversy concerning the nature of this phenomenon, the lack of agreement about the psychological profile, and in many instances the efficacy of treatment. If we are honest with ourselves, we must confess that we are still in the dark as to the fundamental cause of this tantalizing affliction as well as being ignorant as to its logical treatment.

REFERENCES

1. Friedman AP, Mikropoulos HE: Cluster headaches. *Neurology* 1958; 8: 657-659.
2. Kunkle EC, Pfeiffer JB, Wilhoit WM and Hamrick LD: Recurrent brief headache in "cluster" pattern. *Tr AM Neurol A* 1952; 77:240-243.
3. Graham JE, Rogado AZ, Raltman M et al: *Some Physical, Physiological and Psychological Characteristics of Patients with Headache in Background to Migraine* Cochrane AL (ed). London, Heineman, 1970, p. 38-51.
4. Kudrow L, Sutkus BJ: MMPI patterns specificity in primary headache disorders. *Headache* 1979; 19:18-24.
5. Symonds C: A particular variety of headache. *Brain* 1956; 79:217-232.
6. Nieman EA, Hurwitz LJ: Ocular sympathetic palsy in periodic migrainous neuralgia *J Neurol Neurosurg Psychiatry* 1961; 24:369-373.
7. Schiller F: Prophylactic and other treatment for "Histaminic Cluster" or Limited variant of migraine. *JAMA* 1960; 173:1907-1911.
8. Steinhilber RM, Pearson JS, Ruston JG: Some psychological considerations of histaminic cephalgia. *Proc Staff Meet Mayo Coin* 1960; 35, 691-699.
9. Rogado A, Harrison RH, Graham JR: Personality profiles in cluster headache, migraine and normal controls. Presented at the 10th International Congress of World Federation of Neurology, Sept 1973.
10. Ekbom K, Olivarious B: Chronic migrainous neuralgia—diagnostic and therapeutic aspects. *Headache* 1971; 11:97-101.
11. Sjaastad O, Dale I: Evidence for a new (?) treatable headache entity: A preliminary report. *Headache* 1974; 14:105-108.
12. Mathew NT: Indomethacin responsive headache syndromes. *Headache* 1981; 21:147-150.
13. Medina LJ, Diamond S: The clinical link between migraine and cluster headache *Arch Neurol* 1977; 34:470-472.
14. Gilbert GJ: Meniere's syndrome and cluster headache recurrent paryxysmal focal vasodilatation. *JAMA* 1965; 191-691-694.

9
The Relation of Cluster Headache to Migraine

JOHN R. GRAHAM

The question of whether cluster headache is a separate disease entity or a related variant of migraine has been widely debated, especially for the past 20 years since the Ad Hoc Committee of the NINDB[1] placed it under the migraine masthead in its Classification of Headache in 1962. Although a number of positive opinions have been expressed on both sides of the issue, I, for the time being, feel a bit like Omar Khayyam the Tentmaker, who said,

> Myself when young did eagerly frequent
> Doctor and Saint, and heard great argument
> About it and about, but evermore
> Came out by the same door wherein I went[2].

I, too, do not intend to provide an answer to this problem in this chapter but rather to examine with you the means by which we relate some clinical entities to each other or separate them, review the similarities and differences between cluster and migraine headaches and their significance in connection with their possible relationship, and consider factors about host and disease and environment which may be influential in shaping the clinical manifestations of medical disorders and possibly point toward their having either a common or a separate origin.

It is an interesting and important question for us all in the headache field to work on, not only because of its own peculiar scientific fascination but also because cluster headache is a disorder peculiarly favorable for investigative techniques. This is because the cluster patient himself presents a headache-laden side and a headache-free side, periods in which he is susceptible to precipitating stimuli and other periods in which he is immune to them. During attacks he provides ipsilateral supplies of fluid for examination, tears, rhinorrhea, saliva and sweat, as well as general sources of gastric secretions, spinal fluid and blood. If cluster headache proves, in the final analysis, to be a close relative of migraine presenting in a dramatic, exaggerated, "compressed" form, then the solution of its pathophysiology may carry over benefits from its rather rare occurrence to the much larger multitudes suffering with migraine.

The clinical presentation of most diseases is usually the result of many important determining factors. These include the nature of the etiological agent or circumstances or stress; the state of susceptibility, resistance or capacity to respond of the person who is affected; the habits, behavior, culture, education, nationality, race, and inheritance of the host; and the nature of the precipitating and alleviating factors.

It is remarkable that so many syndromes are so clearly similar and well-defined considering the multiplicity of factors which mold the clinical shape of a disease syndrome. It is not surprising to find syndromes with the same etiology which deviate from the standard form in varying degrees. By and large we can identify specific disease entities best if we know their tissue pathology. Without the actual microscopic specific lesion, the next most reliable way of determining relationship between syndromes is a detailed knowledge of their key abnormality of pathophysiology. If there are as yet no specific markers either of tissue structure change or physiologic-biochemical aberration, then, in order to relate syndromes, we have to retreat to grouping of clinical signs and symptoms affecting certain systems in a variety of ways but with less direct evidence that they have a common etiological denominator that makes them relatives.

When we examine these three layers of knowledge about disease relationships we still find many variations in the presentation of diseases due to a *known, common* etiological agent. For instance the great imposter, syphilis, caused by the well known easily identified spirochete, may present itself in a wide variety of clinical forms depending on the duration of infection, the resistance of the host, the tissue affected, and the age and sex of the patient.

The whole group of the lymphomatous diseases may present as fever of unknown origin, weight loss, pain in almost any organ, anemia, bowel obstruction, pericardial effusion, etc.

In the biochemical field the presenting symptoms of well-recognized biochemical errors may vary greatly, such as, hyper- and hypothyroidism, hypoglycemia, hypercalcemia, etc., from one individual to another depending on that person's diet, exercise, activity, mental and emotional status, age and sex.

Before these secret covert markers of a disease entity were recognized, before the spirochete was identified, before the urine of the diabetic was found to be sweet with sugar and the sleepiness of the hyperparathyroid was related to high blood calcium, separation of diseases into certain syndromes depended on clinical observations of the manner, occurrence, location and severity of symptoms, their relations to certain stimuli, on effect in the patient and alleviation by thereapeutic weapons.

We must also recognize that identical etiological agents producing symptoms in a patient may create a variety of changes in blood and other chemistry and physiological reaction depending on the organ currently being affected and the severity of the process; some physiological responses that take place as this specific agent goes to work may represent nonspecific responses by the general stress response systems in the body.

When we bring these thoughts to bear on the problem of the relationship, if any, of migraine to cluster headache we have to admit that as yet we cannot point with certainty to any marker, pathological, physiological or biochemical, which is pathognomonic of either one condition or the other. In the area of greater certainty, pathology, we have precious little matériel at all: some scattered examinations of the water content of temporal vessels during migraine by Wolff[3], some evidence of catechol depletion in temporal arteries during headache by Adams[4], some excessive nesting of mast cells and changes in their granulation in cluster headache by Appenzeller[5] and Pruzinski[6], rare and scattered observations, as yet not shown to be specific for migraine or cluster headache. I do not mean to imply that there is no specific pathology lesion in migraine and/or cluster headache, merely that at the present state of the science, we have not identified it.

When we look for evidence at the level of biochemical or pathophysiological changes, we run into such a host of interesting findings that bear some relation to the migraine or cluster attacks that their very number is beginning to boggle the mind. Each month we find more and more substances and variations in the blood and CSF of migraine and cluster patients, and tissue levels are found to go up or down during the headache experience. To date, however, despite changes in one direction or the other, I feel that we have not reached a state of secure knowledge about any one change or group of changes which identifies them specifically as cause or effect of the syndromes. These changes are possibly associated with different biochemical by-products in varying amounts, depending on which area of the cranium is chiefly involved in the biochemical episode and the physiological state of the patient—depression, anger, arousal, sleep, fatigue, or hormonal imbalance.

A great many interesting variables of biochemical and physiological behavior in relation to migraine and cluster headache have been and will be identified as being above or below normal during attacks. The investigation of these changes is very important since it is through such studies that we may eventually find certain abnormal constellations of biochemical or physiological behavior that eventually shine the light on the essential changes responsible for the clinical condition.

At the present time, however, I do not believe the picture is so clear that we can say that because one of these changes is abnormal in migraine but not in cluster headache the two disorders have no common denominator of etiology. These interesting substances include many vasoactive amines, hormones, neuropeptides, kinins, releasing factors, monoamine oxidases, platelet substances, and neurotransmitters, to mention only a few of the rapidly growing list. In all of the studies which relate to changes in these fascinating and powerful substances in headache sufferers and controls we need to compare carefully the states of the human subjects at the time of their examination; for instance we should discover whether the control has just undergone a stress that has led to headache in the migraine subject.

This brings us to consideration of the clinical manifestations of the two clinical entities on which we must, under current knowledge, base the majority of our decisions about this problematical relationship, if we can make one at all.

The best way to look at the problem on this clinical level is to see how migraine and cluster headache match up with each other in key clinical areas and comment on their similarities and differences. I have selected the following key clinical areas for comparison.

Family history.
Prodromes.
Location.
Ability to shift sides.

Nature of the pain.
Physical manifestations of the presence of headache.
Relation to vascular *vs* nerve pathway distribution.
Accompanying symptoms and signs.
Duration.
Severity.
Pattern of occurrence.
Trigger mechanisms.
Response to therapeutic maneuvers.
Behavior of the patient.
Patient's physique, personality and style of managing stress and achieving goals.
Relation to pregnancy, hypertension and vascular disease.
Age and sex distribution.

Althouth figures on the *familial incidence* of cluster headache and also on the familial occurrence of both cluster and migraine headaches in the same family differ widely in various countries, and in the observations of various investigators, there seems to be no doubt that, in general, the influence of heredity is not as great in cluster headache patients as in those with common migraine. Although examples of cluster headache occurring in brothers, father and son, or mother and son do occur, they tend to be the exception rather than the rule (as in migraine). Although this is a pointer toward a major difference between the two entities, we must remember that even in migraine, family incidence is not 100%. It is probably more like 70%, and it is possible that other factors about the person who has the cluster headache may determine the expression of the genetic trait.

Both the succinct and vague *prodromes* which accompany all classic and some 20% to 30% of common migraines seem to be absent in cluster headache attacks; to be sure, there are a number of instances of cluster patients who also have common migraine and a few with classic migraine, but probably not more than might happen in the population at large. There are rare definite examples of short prodromes of scintillating lights in a migraine pattern immediately preceding cluster headache attacks, but they are very rare. More common are prodromes of autonomic abnormalities like small pupil, drooping eyelid, red conjunctiva, blocked and running nose and ipsilateral tearing definitely preceding the head pain by several minutes and occasionally occurring as the prodromal signs of a subsequent severe headache. This could, of course, suggest that the same etiologic factor creates different signs and symptoms when it acts prodromally in a different territory than the usual migraine terrains.

The *location* of both types of head pain is really quite similar. It tends to follow a vascular distribution rather than a nerve distribution. Its laterality—an important feature among the headaches—is similar to migraine. Also important is the *capacity to shift sides* during an attack, from one attack to another and from one cluster to another, and even to be bilaterally present during the same attack. These features which the two disorders have in common I consider important evidence in favor of a common etiological mechanism.

The *nature of the pain* gets different adjectives from the patients but they may represent chiefly matters of degree of pain. Both steady and throbbing pain are recorded in each condition but words suggesting thalamic pain, pulling, tearing, searing, knifelike, excruciating, are more common in cluster attacks—probably due solely to the greater intensity of the pain. *Excruciating* pain occurs in both entities. It is the rule in cluster and the exception in migraine.

During and sometimes preceding attacks of cluster headache the patient or his spouse may note various *physical manifestations*: "the distended vein" on the forehead, the gray color of the patient (or, rarely, flushed appearance), the small pupil and swelling, drooping eyelid and beginning tears and blocking of the nose. Although these are dramatically noticeable in cluster attacks, close observation will reveal similar findings in miniature at times in common migraine. Stuffed nose is common; smaller orbital fissure is not rare, and slight watering of the eye may be noticed by patient and spouse in common migraine—a change largely of degree.

In both disorders pressure on the swollen vessels may bring superficial and temporary relief, as will injection around the temporal artery by xylocaine. In both conditions surgical interruption of branches of the external carotid may bring relief—usually temporary and partial but occasionally permanent.

Accompanying *systemic signs*, such as nausea, vomiting, diarrhea and diuresis, are certainly much more common in migraine but yet occur occasionally in cluster headache.

The *duration* of given attacks is certainly very much shorter in cluster headache than in common or classic migraine. Rare attacks of cluster headache have been noted to last from eight to 12 hours but this is the great exception for cluster and is the rule for migraine.

The *pattern of occurring* in clusters is certainly characteristic of cluster headache. Clustering of a sort, however, is not uncommon in classic migraine in which small clusters or flurries, are followed by prolonged weeks of freedom. Now we are learning more of "cyclical migraine"—a disorder in which common migraine attacks occur with great frequency for weeks or months and then present equally long periods free of headache. Even tic douloureux comes in bursts or bouts. "Clustering" is not specifically pathognomic of cluster headache.

The *stimuli* which produce cluster and migraine attacks are strikingly similar. Alcohol, nitroglycerine, histamine, let-down in pace and mental activity, cessation of sustained hyperactivity, emotional upset aftermath, sleep—especially REM sleep, certain days of the week, vacation, conclusion of mental or emotional problems are all post-stress, vasodilatory, let-down cessations or arousal activities which seem to have a common effect in the production of both cluster and migraine headaches.

Their *response to therapeutic maneuvers* is also in large part similar. They benefit by ergotamine, methysergide, periactin, steroids, oxygen—agents which usually do not affect other kinds of headache. They differ in response to lithium in that the latter seems very helpful to cluster but apparently not usually to migraine, although our experience in this is not great in migraine.

In our limited experience, but not that of others, it would appear that *pregnancy* is helpful to both cluster and common migraine.

Although the *age* of onset of migraine tends to be earlier in general than that of cluster headache, examples of the latter are appearing more frequently in little children and not uncommonly in teenagers, and continue on into the 70s as in migraine.

The *sex* distribution in cluster is certainly the reverse of that in common migraine, even to the extent that some of the women who have cluster tend to be a bit masculine in their physical appearance and even their mental attitudes.

As time goes by, we in our clinic see more and more patients with headache that is hard to place as to whether it is in the cluster or the migraine group, either by the severity of attacks, the behavior of the patients (which in migraine is hibernation but in cluster is frantic aggressive action), patterns of duration, clustering or grouping —an interesting no-man's land where over time a given patient seems to step from one pattern into another. In one family we have a mother with common migraine, a father with cluster headache, a daughter with both migraine and cluster (both improve with pregnancy), and a son who has common migraine in daily cycles for three months of the year and no headache the rest of the time. And we have the patient who starts with classic migraine and slips over into cluster headaches with all the autonomic fixings, and the girl who has clearly one type or the other at various times and in between has a separate entity with prominent features and responses of both.

One theory we have is that the make-up of the host has quite a lot to do in vascular headache of the migraine type with the pattern of its occurrence. It has been observed that cluster headache patients tend to be tall, athletic, and husky, with a leonine appearance. They strive hard to live up to a "macho" image but have the same emotional needs for support as other people do. The usual migraine patient may have a headache each weekend when relaxation from a tense week takes place. Another person, like many of the "type A" cluster men—have a need to live up to their highly masculine appearance which keeps them at a constant high pitch for a prolonged time, capable until a major let-down renders them vulnerable to a series of attacks arising from their relaxed post-stress state.

A final disquieting thought enters our consideration these days. Perhaps some other undetermined factor besides heredity may play a role in rendering cluster headache patients susceptible to major vascular changes in relation to their state of resistance to stress or immunity, and that such a factor, in addition to the patient's personal life style, may determine the clustering phenomena related to a common causal agent between migraine and cluster. Interesting candidates for such a hidden role are the herpes or other neurologic viruses which lie dormant in key sensory and autonomic ganglia of the head only to be reactivated by stress, fever, sunlight, emotion, physical manipulation and changes in the immune balance within their host.

It seems that the major clinical differences between migraine and cluster headache are matters of timing and severity and probably location of action. In other respects—their vascular involvement, unilaterality, ability to shift sides, response to therapeutic agents and precipitation by similar trigger mechanisms, relation to change in mental and emotional pace—these could well be within the range of possibility of variance in a syndrome based in a common cause but altered by the terrain and life style of the host.

The same pathophysiological process taking place in one patient in the occipital cortex and in another in the forebrain or anterior cranial structures may produce head pain with different timing, severity, chemistry, and clinical signs and symptoms. I must admit, however, that the clinical picture as seen in the active cluster patient during an attack presents a dramatically different picture from that of migraine.

As intimated at the beginning, I bring no certain answer to the problem; but it is often wiser to have no answer (as yet) than a wrong answer. Claude Bernard, the father of the experimental method in science, a very curious man, said in one of his note books: "My philosophy is 'je ne sais pas.' I wish to search for the answers but 'je dors comfortablement sur l'oreiller de 'je ne sais pas'." I sleep comfortably on the pillow of "I don't know." This attitude of keeping an open mind until we have more certain markers to identify etiology of these conditions may be the wisest attitude to preserve.

REFERENCES

1. Ad Hoc Committee on Classification of Headache of the National Institute of Neurological Diseases and Blindness: Classification of Headache. *JAMA* 1962; 179:717–18.
2. Khayyam O. Rubaiyat: Stanza 27 (translated by Edward Fitzgerald). *Familiar Quotations*, John Bartlett, ed 13, Boston, Little Brown, 1955:532a.
3. Wolff HG: *Headache and Other Head Pain*. New York, Oxford University Press, 1948:296–298.
4. Adams CWM: Arterial catecholamine and enzyme histochemistry in migraine. *J Neurol Neurosurg Psychiatry* 1968; 31:50.
5. Appenzeller O, Becker W, Ragas A: Cluster headache, ultrastructural aspects. *Neurology* 1978; 28:371.
6. Prusinski A, Liberski PP: Is the cluster headache local mastocytic diathesis? *Headache* 1979; 19:102.

10
Treatment and Management of Acute Cluster Headache

JAMES R. COUCH, JR.

INTRODUCTION

Cluster headache is one of the most painful "functional" syndromes that exists. The patient with an acute cluster headache suffers with tremendous pain, and then, following cessation of the headaches, lives in mortal fear of the next one. Indeed, more than one account has stated that patients may consider suicide during a cluster headache. Some patients have indicated they are prevented from doing harm to themselves only by the knowledge that the pain is usually self-limited 30 to 120 minutes. Cluster headache patients seek any modality that will produce relief. The therapeutic armamentarium is not large, but several effective approaches are available.

ERGOT PREPARATION

Ergotamine

Ekbom[1] found that ergotamine tartrate was useful in therapy of cluster headache. Subsequently, studies by Symonds[2], Friedman and Mikropoulos[3] and Kudrow[4,5] have investigated this more thoroughly. A number of other authors have also mentioned ergotamine as very effective.

In order to be effective, ergotamine must be used early in the attack. Once the attack is well established, effectiveness declines significantly[5]. Kudrow suggests that the oral route of administration is not suitable since gastroparesis may accompany the cluster headache thus slowing absorption and slowing onset of therapeutic effect[5]. Use of suppositories is not suitable for many patients as the cluster headache patient is often nervous, irritable and developing a terror of the coming pain. Cluster headache patients usually find that they have to be up and moving and cannot lie down. This may make administration and retention of the suppository difficult.

The sublingual form of ergotamine is probably the most effective way of administering the drug. Intranasal sprays have been used in Europe, but are not available in this country.

The dose of ergotamine that may be used is 1 to 2 mg at the onset of the cluster headache and then the dose may be repeated 15 to 30 minutes later and, if necessary, in another 15 to 30 minutes.

Ergotamine had been reported to be effective in 50 to 85% of subjects. Friedman and Mikropoulos[3] found that ergotamine was successful as a symptomatic therapy 85% of the time. Kudrow[4,5] has reported that ergotamine was successful in aborting eight of ten consecutive cluster headaches in 70% of a group of 50 patients. This would generally agree with this author's experience in the use of ergotamine for patients with cluster headache.

The onset of the effect of sublingual ergotamine is somewhat variable. Kudrow found that 35% of his subjects reported relief in four to nine minutes and 65% by ten to 15 minutes[4]. Some subjects with headaches that are characteristically 15 to 30 minutes in duration are unsure if there is a therapeutic effect, but take the medication anyway as it makes them feel they are doing something to combat the intense pain.

While ergotamine usually aborts the headache, a significant minority of patients claim the ergotamine simply delays the headache. These find that ergotamine will delay the onset of the headache by one to several hours, but the feeling of vague discomfort that precedes the cluster headache remains. The patient then feels he must keep repeating the ergotamine or go on to have the headache before this discomfort clears.

Ergotamine has a number of side effects which limit its use in a significant number of patients. The major side effects are: (1) nausea and vomiting, (2) coronary artery spasm with chest pain, (3) muscle cramps, (4) cyanosis and paresthesias of extremities, (5) intermittent claudication, (6) mental clouding, and (7) peripheral neuropathy[6,7,8]. Nausea, vomiting, or muscle cramping may occur at low or high doses. Arterial spasm is a side effect usually seen only at the higher doses; however, occasional subjects may develop angina or acrocyanosis on low doses of ergotamine. Intermittent claudication and mental clouding have been reported for large doses.

Tolerance and habituation to ergotamine have been noted in several reports[6-9]. While most of these have dealt with ergotamine abuse in migraine, Peters and Horton described 17 patients with cluster headache who abused ergotamine[8]. Only eight of these had toxic reactions to ergotamine and the toxic reactions were not strictly dose related. One patient had taken 13,140 mg of ergotamine over a two year period and manifested only intermittent claudcation of the legs as a toxic effect of ergotamine.

The pharmacology of ergotamine is complex. Ergotamine has effects primarily on smooth muscle and on neural systems employing biogenic amines as neurotransmitters. Fozard has reviewed the pharmacology of ergot compounds and finds that the following five effects may have relevance as to the therapeutic action of ergotamine[10]. At low doses, ergotamine will produce (1) sensitization of smooth muscle to sympathetic stimulation, (2) peripheral vasoconstriction, (3) antagonism of vasoconstrictor responses to serotonin. At higher doses, Ergotamine will produce: (4) inhibition of pulmonary spasmogen release, and (5) inhibition of reuptake of monamines at nerve endings.

Present theory of causation of cluster headache by painful vasodilatation would suggest that the vasoconstrictive action of ergotamine is the major therapeutic one in cluster headache. Effects (1) and (5) above would enhance this constrictive effect and enhance the therapeutic and toxic potential. The issue is not completely settled, however, since Hachinski, et al.[11] found no effect of ergotamine on cerebral circulation at therapeutic doses.

Dihydroergotamine (DHE)

DHE is available only as an injectable agent. It can be used for aborting cluster headache by giving a 1 mg injection. The patient must be trained to given himself injections and be able to prepare the injection as the prodrome of the headache develops. This limits the usefulness of DHE very significantly. Repetition of dose is also a problem as the patient would have to prepare a repeat dose in the midst of the pain of the cluster headache.

The pharmacology of DHE is similar to that for ergotamine. Vasoconstriction is probably the major pharmacologic effect that relates to its therapeutic role in cluster headache. The dose schedule for DHE is similar to that for Ergotamine. Abuse of DHE was documented by Horton and Peters[8].

OXYGEN

Horton[12] noted that oxygen inhalation was successful in relieving cluster headache in some patients. Friedman and Mikropoulos[3] supported this observation, but noted that oxygen was not as effective as ergotamine. Graham likewise found some beneficial effect of oxygen inhalation in occasional patients[13].

Kudrow[4] carried out a recent study of oxygen inhalation in comparison to ergotamine therapy that has helped establish this modality as a major therapeutic approach to cluster headache. In a pilot study, 33 subjects with episodic cluster headache and 19 patients with chronic cluster headache participated (45 males, 7 females). These subjects treated ten consecutive attakcs with oxygen inhalation at seven liters per minute. A "treatment success" was defined as cessation of pain within 15 minutes for 7 of the 10 attacks of cluster headache. About 75% of the subjects were treatment successes as defined above.

In a subsequent study of 50 patients, a similar format was used to test effectiveness of oxygen inhalation against that of sublinqual ergotamine[5]. Ergotamine or oxygen was given at the onset of the cluster headache. Ergotamine could be repeated at 15 and 30 minutes if necessary. The subjects were divided into two groups of 25. One group received oxygen followed by ergotamine while the other received the agents in reverse order. Overall, 82% of subjects aborted eight of ten cluster headache with oxygen, while with ergotamine, 70% of subjects had the same level of response. The differences between oxygen and Ergotamine therapy were not significant.

Kudrow found that of subjects that responded to oxygen, 46% could abort the cluster headache in four to six minutes and another 40% within 12 minutes. The comparative response to Ergotamine was that 29% of responders had relief in six minutes and an additional 45% by 12 minutes.

The author's experience with oxygen therapy is similar to that reported above. A majority of patients respond well to oxygen; however, some patients find that the headache may recur within a short time and require repeat administration of oxygen. As noted above for ergotamine, some patients find that oxygen delays, but does not abort the headache and the headaches will finally commence.

The mechanism of action of oxygen is open to speculation. Oxygen will produce cerebral vasoconstriction in the normal situation. Investigating cerebral blood flow in cluster headache patients, Sakai and Meyer found there was hyperresponsiveness to oxygen inhalation during a cluster headache with a greater than usual fall in cerebral blood flow following oxygen inhalation[12,14]. Between headaches responsiveness of the cerebral circulation to oxygen was normal[13]. Thus oxygen, like ergotamine, may exert its effect by producing a transient cerebral vasoconstriction and this effect is intensified by a hyperresponsiveness of the cerebral circulation to oxygen during the headache.

OTHER THERAPIES FOR ACUTE CLUSTER HEADACHE

Steroids

Use of steroids in cluster headache belongs, for the most part, under prophylactic therapy. The response to steroids may be so dramatic at times that this modality could be considered a therapy for the acute headache. Jammes[16] reported that a single dose of 30 mg of prednisone produced complete relief for ten or more days in 16 of 17 patients in an uncontrolled study. While steroids should not, in most cases, be considered as an acute treatment, this might be an alternative consideration if other modalities have failed.

Intranasal Cocaine

The similarity of pain intensity and location for cluster headache and Sluder's sphenopalatine ganglion neuralgia has led investigators to consider the same treatment for cluster headache as was found effective for Sluder's neuralgia. (See Barre[17] for discussion). Sluder described application of cocaine soaked pledgets to the region of the sphenopalatine ganglia for relief of sphenopalatine neuralgia (cited from Barre[17]). Schiller reported on this type of therapy, finding that 12 of 25 subjects had good results with relief of headache[18]. Barre attempted a similar protocol with subjects administering intranasal application of a 10% cocaine solution to the area of the sphenopalatine ganglion[17]. Patients were given a 10% cocaine solution and told to administer 0.33 to 0.5 cc via a nasal dropper. Patients were told to lie supine with the head tilted backward towards the floor at 30° and turned to the side of the headache. Administration was allowed twice in a 5 hour period. Of 12 subjects, 11 reported 80% relief within 2½ minutes. In two cases, a miotic pupil that had developed with the headache reverted to normal within two minutes.

The amount of relief obtained here suggests that cluster headache may relate to reflex circuits that involve the nasal mucosa and its underlying structures. On the other hand, Barre points out that there is rapid systemic absorption of cocaine through the nasal mucosa[17] and the possibility of the results being related to a systemic effect of cocaine must be considered.

This study does suggest cocaine may be an agent with promise in treatment of cluster headache. Nevertheless, development of this therapeutic agent may be severely limited by the abuse potential.

Analgesics and Narcotics

The patients who have cluster headache of longer duration frequently request additional analgesic medication for relief from the pain. Additionally, during a cycle of frequent and severe cluster headache, some patients will manifest a residual soreness and tenderness in the area of the headache between the actual cluster headaches. Propoxyphene and codeine preparations are usually useful in this group of patients. Occasionally, pentozacine or meperidine might be considered. In general, since the pain is self-limited and since there is gastroparesis associated with the cluster headache, the administration of oral pain medication is futile because no medication will reach the blood stream in adequate levels until the headache is almost terminated. Patients suffering with the pain of the cluster headache, however, often prefer to feel as if they are doing something to combat the pain and a significant relief related to placebo effect must be considered. In general, the least habituating agent should be employed because of the abuse potential.

CONCLUSION

The agents that are effective in acute cluster headache all have in common the ability to produce vasoconstriction in the cranial or cerebral circulation. Although the mechanism of cluster headache is still only speculative, the concept of painful vasodilatation around the orbit continues to be the major hypothesis of pathogenesis for this condition. From this hypothesis, it can be postulated that vasoconstrictors would produce relief and this has been the case.

The mainstays of acute therapy of cluster headache are ergotamine given by a route that bypasses the stomach and oxygen administration. There may be a role for intranasal cocaine, but the abuse potential will likely limit the use of this modality. Future research into other local agents that produce vasoconstriction in the nasal mucosa may be useful in terms of elucidating pathogenetic mechanisms and providing new approaches for relief in this very painful condition.

REFERENCES

1. Ekbom K: A clinical comparison of cluster headache and migraine. *Acta Neurol Scand* 1970; 41(suppl):1-48.
2. Symonds SC: A particular variety of headache. *Brain* 1956; 79:217-232.
3. Friedman AP, Mikropoulos HE: Cluster headaches. *Neurology* 1958; 8:653-663.
4. Kudrow L: Response of cluster headache attacks to oxygen inhalation. *Headache* 1981; 21:1-4.
5. Kudrow L: *Cluster Headache, Mechanisms and Management*, New York, Oxford University Press, 1980.
6. Friedman AP, Brazil P, vonStorch TJC: Ergotamine tolerance in patients with migraine. *JAMA* 1955; 157:881-884.
7. Peters GA, Horton BT: Headache: With special reference to the excessive use of ergotamine preparations and withdrawal effects. *Proc Staff Meet Mayo Clin* 1951; 26:153-161.
8. Horton BT, Peters GA: Clinical manifestations of excessive use of ergotamine preparations and management of withdrawal effects: Report of 52 cases. Headache 1963; 2:214-227.
9. Andersson PG: Ergotamine headache. *Headache* 1975; 15:118-121.
10. Fozard JR: The animal pharmacology of drugs used in the treatment of migraine. *J Pharm Pharmacol* 1975; 27:297-321.
11. Hachinski V, Norris JW, Edmeads J, Cooper PW: Ergotamine and cerebral blood flow. Stroke 1978; 9:594-596.
12. Horton BT: Histaminic cephalgia. *J Lancet* 1952; 72:92-98.
13. Graham JR: Cluster headache. *Headache* 1972; 11:175-185.
14. Sakai F, Meyer JS: Abnormal cerebrovascular reactivity in patients with migraine and cluster headaches. *Headache* 1979; 19:257-266.
15. Amano T, Meyer JS: Prostaglandin inhibition and cerebrovascular control in patients with headache. *Headache* 1982; 22:52-59.
16. Jammes JL: The treatment of cluster headaches with Prednisone. *Dis Nerv Syst* 1975; 36:375-376.

17. Barre F: Cocaine as an abortive agent in cluster headache. *Headache* 1982; 22:69-73.
18. Schiller F: Prophylactic and other treatment for "histaminic," "cluster," or "limited" variant of migraine. *JAMA* 1960; 173:87-91.

11
Prophylactic Pharmacotherapy of Cluster Headache

NINAN T. MATHEW

Prophylactic use of pharmacotherapeutic agents on a daily basis during the cluster periods has come to be accepted as the most effective means of managing cluster headache. The rationale of using prophylactic medications breaks down as follows:

1. Attacks of cluster headaches are too short-lived for abortive medications to take effect in a significant number of patients. The evaluation of abortive medications during acute attacks becomes difficult because of the "natural self-limiting duration" of each attack.
2. In some patients ergotamine and oxygen may not fully abort the attacks, but simply delay it, with the headache recurring within a short time and requiring repeat administration of agents.
3. A large number of attacks in a given day results in overmedication, especially if one uses ergotamine or a narcotic pain medication.
4. If the cluster period is not stopped early, the suffering may continue for months.

The above reasons have led to the search for pharmacotherapeutic agents which can be used on a daily basis during the cluster period. These medications can be classified into those which can be beneficially used and those with questionable value. The most beneficial agents are: (1) ergotamine tartrate,[1] (2) methysergide maleate,[2-11] (3) corticosteroids,[11-16] (4) lithium carbonate,[17-21] (5) indomethacin,[22,23] and (6) BC105[24,25].

There are a number of other medications which have been and are being used in the prophylaxis of cluster headache whose beneficial effects are of questionable value. These include: (1) Histamine desensitization,[26-29] (2) Chlorpromazine,[30] (3) Beta blockers, (4) Tricyclic antidepressants, and (5) Phenyl propanolamine (active ingredient in "Sinutab").[31]

PRINCIPALS OF PROPHYLACTIC PHARMACO-THERAPY

The principles of prophylactic pharmacotherapy during cluster headache are:

1. To start the medications early in the cluster period.
2. To use the medications daily until the patient is free of headache for at least two weeks.
3. Taper the medications gradually rather than abruptly withdrawing them.
4. Restart the medications at the beginning of the next cluster period.
5. Explain the side effects of all the medications used.

It is unrealistic to expect a 100% prevention of all attacks during the cluster period with the presently available agents. Reduced frequency, severity and duration of attacks should be weighed against the hazards of overmedication. Symptomatic or abortive medications can be used in the event of a breakthrough of attacks.

SELECTION OF PROPHYLACTIC MEDICATION REGIMENS

Each physician and clinic establishes its own treatment regimens and criteria of selection of patients for various medications. Our own criteria depend on: (1) Previous response to prior prophylactic medications, (2) Adverse reactions to prior medications, (3) Presence of contraindications for using a particular medication, (4) Type of cluster headache, (5) Age of patient, (6) Frequency of attacks, (7) Timing of the attacks eg: nocturnal *vs* diurnal, and (8) Expected length of the cluster periods already passed before the prophylactic treatment could be initiated.

It is helpful to examine the individual medications used in the prophylaxis of cluster headache.

Ergotamine

Ergotamine was first used prophylactically by K. A. Ekbom in 1947 who reported success in 13 out of 16 patients in whom he used 2 mg. of ergotamine tartrate orally two to three times a day. While ergotamine has to be used sublingually, parenterally, or as inhalation for effective abortive treatment, it can be used successfully via oral route in prophylactic treatment. Our practice is to use 1 mg twice a day of ergotamine irrespective of the occurance of headache and not to use any extra ergotamine for abortive therapy, but to use oxygen inhalation for treatment of individual attacks. Ergotamine is combined with one of the other prophylactic agents, such as methysergide, prednisone, or lithium. The PM dose of ergotamine is usually given at bed time, in order to help prevent nocturnal attacks. An occasional patient with severe or multiple nocturnal attacks may require an additional dose of ergotamine at night.

Complications and contraindications of ergotamine therapy should always be kept in mind. Because of the self-limiting nature of episodic cluster headache long term toxicity is rarely seen in patients with episodic cluster headache. It is the impression of many experienced clinicians that ergotamine rebound headache is not usually seen in cluster headache patients.

Methysergide

Methysergide has potent antiserotonin effects and it antagonizes serotonin induced vasoconstriction of the internal carotid arterial system by both competitive and noncompetitive mechanisms. Sicuteri[2] initiated the use of methysergide in the prophylactic treatment of cluster headache. A number of studies[3-11] have confirmed its value as a prophylactic agent and the overall success rate is about 70%.

Table I (reproduced from Kudrow 1980[16]) summarizes the experience with methysergide.

Methysergide is most effective in younger patients with episodic cluster headache[16]. There appears to be a relative loss of effectiveness in subsequent cluster periods in the same individual.[10,11]

Table 1   Results of Methysergide Maintenance Therapy in
Cluster Headache

Author(s)	Year	No. of patients	Good to excellent results N (%)
Sicuteri	1959	2	2(100)
Heyck	1960	8	8(100)
Friedman	1960	3	2(67)
Graham	1960	20	16(80)
Bergouignan and Seihean	1960	3	3(100)
Friedman and Losin	1961	21	15(71)
Harris	1961	5	5(100)
Hale and Reed	1962	8	3(38)
Lovshin	1963	159	110(69)
Kudrow	1978	77	50(65)

Resistance to treatment often develops after prior treatment of several periods. Our practice is to start with 1 tab the first day and increase the dosage by 1 tab daily until a four times a day dosage is reached. Acute side effects can be minimized to a great degree by gradual increase in the dosage.

Methysergide has no place in the abortive treatment of cluster headache nor is it very useful in chronic cluster headache. Prolonged therapy is required in chronic cluster headache and in an occasional case of chronic cluster headache responsive to methysergide, the therapy may have to be interrupted every three to four months.

Side Effects of Methysergide

Short term

1. About 40% of the patients experience side effects initially which will subside after some days or weeks; these are abdominal discomfort, nausea, vomiting, and muscle cramps or muscle aches.
2. Less common side effects are: insomnia, depression, sensation of swelling in the face and throat, increase in the venules over the nose and cheeks, and weight gain.
3. Ten percent have to discontinue medication because of unpleasant continuing side effects. These include intermittent claudication or other symptoms and signs of peripheral ischemia or angina pectoris. These are reversible.

Long Term

More serious long term side effects are retroperitoneal fibrosis, pleural fibrosis, pulmonary fibrosis, or cardiac valvular fibrosis.[32-34] The fibrotic complications are reversible and resolve completely once the treatment is ceased. The development of fibrotic changes depend on the length of continuous treatment. Fibrotic complications of methysergide may well be the result of its serotoninlike action. Methysergide induces valvular fibrosis resembling that seen in carcinoid syndrome.

Precautions

1.   *Drug holiday* for two months after continuous treatment for four months.
2.   Periodic BUN and creatinin levels, and IVP and echocardiogram at least once a year if the patient is on prolonged treatment.

Contraindications

1.   Peripheral vascular disease, coronary disease, hypertension, and thrombophlebitis; because of the vasoconstrictive effect.
2.   Active peptic ulcer; methysergide increases gastric acid secretion.

Corticosteroids

The use of steroids in cluster headache was first introduced by Horton[35]. Friedman and Mikropoulos[27] did not find corticosteroids useful, while MacNeal[12] and Graham[14] reported beneficial effects. The first controlled study was that of James[13] in 1975 who found prednisone was an effective alternate treatment for cluster headache patients who were resistant to ergotamine and methysergide. Kudrow[11,16] reported marked relief for cluster headache in 76.6% and partial improvement in 11.7% of patients on prednisone treatment for episodic cluster headache which was resistant to methysergide. Responsiveness in chronic cluster headache was less significant; 40% showing marked improvement and 33% showing partial improvement. Couch and Zeigler[15] used prednisone 10 to 80 mg per day in 19 patients. Fourteen of the 19 patients (73%) showed greater than 50% improvement and 11 or 58% had 100% relief. The remaining five had less than 50% improvement. Recurrence of cluster headache was noted in 79% when prednisone was tapered down to between 10 to 20 mg per day. They concluded that prednisone is effective for relief of cluster headache, but warned of the recurrence when dosage is reduced.

The mechanism of action of steroids in cluster headache is speculative. Suppression of the inflammatory response to released humoral agents or suppression of the synthesis of the humoral agents themselves are two possibilities. Because of the recurrence of headaches on discontinuation of steroids, it is obvious that the basic mechanisms are only temporarily suppressed.

Kudrow[16] uses steroids as the first line medication for people between the ages of 35 to 50, as he feels that their response to methysergide is poor. While it is true that younger patients may respond better to methysergide, it is difficult to set any absolute age limit while choosing a prophylactic therapy. Dosage varies from clinic to clinic, we give 40 mg (20mg BID) for approximately two weeks and taper the dose to discontinue them in 3 weeks.

The side effect of steroids are numerous and patients should be thoroughly warned about them. Risks of long term steroids are too severe to justify its prolonged use in chronic cluster headache.

Lithium Carbonate

The indications for lithium carbonate are 1) Chronic cluster headache, 2) Episodic cluster headache resistant to other medications, and 3) Cyclical migraine.

History

Cyclic affective disorders such as manic-depressive psychosis have been found to respond to lithium therapy. Since cluster headache occurs cyclically, Ekbom[17] introduced the use of lithium in cluster headache. Its effect was later confirmed by Kudrow[18], Mathew[19], and Savoldi[20] et al.

Lithium salts were used in the treatment as a sedative and an anticonvulsant in the nineteenth century. The ill-advised use of lithium as a salt substitute for cardiac and the chronically ill patients in the 1940s led to several reports of severe toxic reactions and death, and to considerable notoriety concerning lithium within the medical profession.

Biological Effects

Lithium is a mood stabilizing agent and not a sedative, depressant or euphoriant. The effect on biological membranes is suspected as the main mechanism of action. Lithium ion has a relatively small gradient of distribution across biological membranes, unlike sodium and potassium. While it can replace sodium in supporting single action potential in a nerve cell, it is not an adequate "substrate" for sodium pump and it cannot, therefore, maintain membrane potentials.

Lithium is readily absorbed from the gastrointestinal (GI) tract, reaches a peak plasma concentration in two to four hours, and crosses the blood brain barrier slowly. Ninety-five percent of the drugs are excreted in urine. There is an initial rapid phase of excretion followed by a slower phase lasting up to 14 days. Since 80% of the filtered sodium is reabsorbed by renal tubules, lithium clearance by the kidneys is about 20% that of creatinine. Sodium loading produces a small enhancement for lithium excretion, but sodium depletion promotes a clinically important degree of retention of lithium. Therefore, concomitant use of sodium depleting diuretics should be avoided.

Mechanism of Action of Lithium in Cluster Headache

It has been suggested that a feature common to all disorders responding to lithium therapy is a cyclic, periodic or episodic pattern and cluster headache certainly falls in that category. Other actions of lithium which may be of importance in relation to cluster headache are inhibition of the effect of prolactin on prostaglandin biosynthesis, its effect on monoamines, cyclic adenosine monophosphate (AMP), platelets, and sleep. Cluster headaches are shown to occur in relation to REM sleep[36]. Lithium reduces the mean percentage of REM sleep period, and increases latency of the first REM period in depressed patients.[37,38] Recently lithium has been shown to stabilize serotonin neurotransmission within the CNS,[39] possibly explaining its mode of action in this disorder.

Dosage and Duration of Treatment

Most patients require only 600 to 1200 mgs of lithium administration in divided dosage. Because of its short half-life, divided daily doses are recommended. Lithium levels are obtained after six or seven days initially and at least once a month thereafter.

Duration of treatment varies with the type of headache condition. For episodic cluster headache the treatment is discontinued if the patient remains free of headache for two weeks consecutively. For the chronic variety of cluster headache the lithium treatment may have to be long-term under careful supervision.

The following summarizes the long-term experience with lithium at our clinic. Ekbom's observations[21] were similar.

1. Most lithium responders will benefit from a daily dose of 600 to 900 mg and only an occasional patient will require greater amounts.
2. The serum level required for effective therapeutic response is usually 0.4–0.8 mEq/L which is less than that recommended in cases of manic-depressive psychoses.
3. Patients who improve on lithium experience dramatic relief within the first week.
4. Chronic cluster headache patients appear to be more responsive to lithium than those with episodic patterns.
5. Episodic patients having a prolonged cluster period or who are resistant to other prophylactic medications appear to respond better than typical episodic types.
6. Approximately 60% of responders from the chronic group experience bursts of short cluster periods during lithium maintenance. These attacks are usually less severe and of shorter duration.
7. Approximately 20% of chronic cluster responders became episodic.
8. Approximately 40% of all cluster patients maintained on lithium require concomitant ergotamine prophylaxis for complete relief.
9. As months go by there may be a tendency for the effect to wane and there have been cases which became resistant to lithium after a treatment period of 18 to 24 months.
10. Lithium does not appear to prevent alcohol-induced cluster attacks.

Side Effects and Monitoring

1. *Neurotoxic*: Tremor (propranolol antidote), lethargy, slurring, blurred vision, confusion, nystagmus and ataxia, extrapyramidal signs and seizures if toxic level is reached. Excessive lithium levels and neurotoxicity can develop early in patient on poor salt diet and/or diuretics.
2. *Thyroid*:
    a. Nontender thyroid enlargement. It is reversible on discontinuation of lithium.
    b. Hypothyroidism in 5%, more in females.
    c. Clinical awareness is important to detect hypothyroidism (fatigue, constipation, menstrual irregularities, cold intolerance).

    d. TSH, T3, T4, prior to therapy and at six month intervals, especially in women.

    e. Maintain lithium.

3. *Renal*: Initially there is some sodium retention and edema formation. Polyuria, polydipsia, and nephrogenic diabetes insipidus may occur. Lithium tends to block the action of antidiuretic hormone (ADH) on the renal tubules. Irreversible glomerular sclerosis and tubular fibrosis have been reported.[40,41]

    Therefore, renal monitoring for patients on lithium therapy at least once in six months is recommended. This consists of:

    1. Urine concentration following 12 hour dehydration

        a. >600 mOsm/kg

        b. >1.018 specific gravity

    2. $C_{cr} = \dfrac{(140 - age)(wt,kg)}{72 \times S_{cr}\,(mg/100\ ml)}$ (15% less in females)

    3. Routine urinalysis

4. *Hematologic*:

    a. Reversible polymorhonuclear leucocytosis which should not be mistaken for occult infection.

    b. Anecdotal reports of increased incidence of acute leukemia, controversial at present. The bulk of available evidence weighs against lithium as a cause of leukemia.

    c. Advisable to obtain a complete blood count prior to initiating lithium therapy, and once or twice a year afterwards.

5. *Drug interactions*: anecdotal reports that phenytoxin may potentiate lithium-induced side effects.

6. *Sleep disorders*:

    a. Increases the amount of slow wave sleep and suppresses REM to some degree.

    b. Increases the changes of sleep walking (somnambulism) if combined with antipsychotic drugs.

7. *Cardiac*:

    a. T-wave flattening (about 50% of patients). It is a benign change.

    b. Sinus node dysfunction—three cases reported. Exercise tolerance unaffected—generally considered extremely rare.

    c. Relatively safe drug overall from a cardiac point of view.

8. *Dermatologic*:

    a. Acne like eruptions

    b. Hyperkerotic papuls, cutaneous ulcers, thinning of the hair

    c. Precipitation and aggravation of psoriasis

9. *Pregnancy*:
   a. Congenital cardiac malformation in newborn of mothers taking lithium, especially Ebstein's malformation.
   b. Neonatal goiter
   c. CNS depression in infants
   d. Hypotonia in infants

The relationship between the doses of a drug required to produce undesired and desired effects is termed its therapeutic index or margin of safety. Because of the low therapeutic index for lithium, concentration in plasmas must be determined periodically. The recommended therapeutic range for manic depressive is 0.6 to 15 mEq/L. It is our experience that patients with cluster headache required (0.4 to 0.8 mEq/L) of serum lithium levels for adequate therapeutic response. These concentrates refer to blood samples obtained ten to two hours after the last dose of the day.

Since lithium is secreted in human milk, women on lithium should not breast feed infants.

Indomethacin

Sjaastad[42] has recently reviewed the cases of chronic paroxysmal hemicrania which continue to appear to be a variant of cluster headache with a remarkable responsivity to Indomethacin. Indomethacin completely eliminates the attacks and according to Sjaastad it is essential for the diagnosis. The dosage varies from 12.5 to 250 mg per day. We generally use 50mg three times a day. The benefit usually appears in 48 hours. Tolerance to indomethacin has not yet been observed with a follow up of five months to 6½ years.[42]

Side Effects: Side effects are developed by 35%.
1. Gastric irritation, nausea, vomiting, activation of peptic ulcer, melena, occult blood loss, anemia
2. Rarely pancreatitis, hepatitis, jaundice
3. Headache in 25 to 50%, frontal
4. Dizziness, occasional mental confusion
5. Severe psychosis has occurred
6. Hypersensitivity skin reactions
7. Benign intracranial hypertension has been reported

MEDICATIONS OF QUESTIONABLE VALUE
IN CLUSTER HEADACHE

A comprehensive review of the current status of Histamine desentization is given by Campbell[43] and hence will not be discussed here.

Chlorpromazine was reported as a useful drug by Caviness and O'Brien,[30] but there has been no further published data on chlorpromazine in cluster headache. From personal exchange of information among physicians interested in this field, chlorpromazine does not appear to be useful.

Medications such as propranolol and amitriptyline which are found to be useful in the prophylactic treatment of migraines and mixed vascular-muscle contraction headache, are found to be not especially effective in the prophylactic treatment of cluster headaches. It should be pointed out that during cluster headaches, there is significant bradycardia,[44] and this should be borne in mind when one prescribes propranolol. It is our practice not to use propranolol or amitriptyline in case of cluster headache.

Finally the physician may have to combine the art of medicine and the science of medicine in the management of this most fascinating of human ailments. The choice of drugs and the length of treatment prescribed are entirely left to the individual physicians experience, convictions and reasoning. Our own regimen is to use combinations of ergotamine prophylaxis with either sansert or prednisone in episodic cluster headache and lithium in chronic cluster headache. Management of the treatment-resistant patients remains a major issue, and is discussed elsewhere in this book.

REFERENCES

1. Ekbom, KA: Ergotamine tartrate orally in Horton's "histaminic cephalgia" (also called Harris's "ciliary neuralgia"): A new method of treatment. *Acta Psychiat Scand* 1974; 46(suppl):106-113.
2. Sicuteri F: Prophylactic and therapeutic properties of 1-methyl-lysergic acid butanolamide in migraine: preliminary report. *Int Arch Allergy appl Immunol* 1959; 15:300-7.
3. Heyck H: Serotonin antagonists in the therapy of migraine and Bing's erythroprosopalgia or Horton's syndrome. *Schwiez med Wochenschr* 1960; 90:203-9.
4. Friedman AP: Clinical observations with 1-methyl-lysergic acid butanolamide (UML-491) in vascular headache. *Angiology* 1960; 11:364-6.

5. Graham JR: Cardiac and pulmonary fibrosis during methysergide therapy for headaches. *Amer J Med* 1967; 245:23-34.

6. Bergouignan M, Seilhean A: The place of anti-serotonins in the treatment of migraine and vasomotor headache. *Presse med* 1960; 68:2176-8.

7. Friedman AP, Losin S: Evaluation of UML-491 in treatment of vascular headaches: an analysis of the effects of 1-methy-d-lysergic acid (+) butanolamide bimaleate (methysergide). *Arch Neurol* 1961; 4:241-5.

8. Harris W: Ciliary (Migrainous) neuralgia and its treatment. *Br Med J* 1936; 1:457.

9. Hale AF, Reed AF: Prophylaxis of frequent vascular headache with methysergide. *Amer J Med* 1962; 243:942-152.

10. Lovshin LL: Treatment of histaminic cephalgia with methysergide (UML-491). *Dis Nerv Syst* 1963; 24:3-7.

11. Kudrow L: Comparative results of prednisone, methysergide, and lithium therapy in cluster headache. In Green R (ed): *Current Concepts in Migraine Research* New York, Raven Press, 1978, pp 156-63.

12. MacNeal PS: Useful therapeutic approaches to the patient with "problem headache". *Headache* 1975; 14:186-9.

13. Jammes JL: The treatment of cluster headache with prednisone. *Dis Nerv Syst* 1975; 36, 375-6.

14. Graham JR: Cluster headache, in Appenzeller O: *Pathogenesis and Treatment of Headache*. New York, Spectrum Publications, 1976.

15. Couch JR, Ziegler DK: Prednisone Therapy for cluster headache—*Headache* 1978; 18:219-221.

16. Kudrow L: *Cluster Headache. Mechanisms and Management*, Oxford, Oxford Medical Publications, 1980, pp. 127-154.

17. Ekbom K: Litium vid kroniska symptom av cluster headache. Preliminart Meddelande *Pousc Med* 1974; 19:148-56.

18. Kudrow L: Lithium prophylaxis for chronic cluster headache. *Headache* 1977; 17:15-18.

19. Mathew NT: Clinical subtypes of cluster headache and response to lithium therapy. *Headache* 1978; 18, 26-30.

20. Savoldi F, Nappi G, Bono G: Lithium salts in treatment of idiopathic headaches and of facial pain syndromes, in Pinelli P (ed) *Proceedings of the Polish-Italian Meeting of Neurology*, Varenna, June 1978.

21. Ekbom K: Lithium for cluster headache: Review of the leterature and prilimanary results of long term treatment. *Headache* 1981; 12:132-139.

22. Sjaastad O, Dale I: A new (?) clinical headache entity "Chronic Paroxysmal Hemicrania." *Acta Neurol Scand* 1976; 43:150-59.

23. Mathew NT: Indomethacin responsive Headache Syndrome, *Headache* 1981; 21:147-150.

24. Ekbom K: Prophylactic treatment of cluster headache with a new serotonin antagonist, BC 105. *Acta Neurol Scand* 1969; 45:601-10.

25. Sicuteri F, Franchi G, and Del Bianco PL: An antaminic drug BC 105, in the prophylaxis of migraine. *Int Arch Allergy* 1967; 31:78-93.

26. Horton BT, McLean AR, Craig W MCK: The use of histamine in the treatment of specific types of headache. *Proc Staff Meet Mayo Clin* 1939; 14:257.

27. Friedman AP, Mikropoulos HE: Cluster Headache. *Neurology* 1958; 8:63.

28. Kunkel EC, Pfeiffer JB Jr, Wilhoit WM, et al: Recurrent brief headache in cluster pattern. *Tr Am Neurol A* 1952; 77:240.

29. Symonds CA: Particular variety of headache. *Brain* 1956; 79:217.

30. Caviness VS JR., and O'Brien P: Cluster Headache response to chlorpromazine. *Headache* 1980; 20:128-131.

31. Cohen KL: "Sinutabs" for cluster headache. *New Engl J Med* 1980; 303: 107-108.

32. Graham JR: Possible renal complications of Sansert (methysergide) therapy for headache. *Headache* 1965; 5:12-13.

33. Graham JR, Parnes LR: Possible cardiac and reno-vascular complications of Sansert therapy. *Headache* 1965; 5:14-18.

34. Graham JR: Cardiac and pulmonary fibrosis during methysergide therapy for headaches. *Amer J Med* 1967; 245:23-34.

35. Horton BT: Histamine cephalgia. *J Lancet* 1952; 72:92.

36. Dexter JD, Weitzman ED: The relatinship of nocturnal headaches to sleep stage patterns. *Neurology* 1970; 20:513-518.

37. Kupfer DJ, Wyatt RJ, Greenspan K et al: Lithium carbonate and sleep in affective illness. *Arch Gen Psychiat* 1970; 23:35-40.

38. Mendels J, Chernik DA: The effect of Lithium Carbonate on the sleep of Depressed Patients. *Int Pharmaco-Psychiat* 1973; 8:184-192.

39. Ireiser SL: Lithium increases serotomin release and decreases serotomin reception. *Hippolanpus Science* 1981; 213:1529-1531.

40. Jenner FA: Lithium an question of Kidney damage. *Arch Gen Psych* 1979; 36:888-890.

41. Chan WY et al: Lithium nephrotoxicity: A review. *Ann Clin Lab Sci* 1981; 11:343-349.

42. Sjaastad O, et al: Chronic paroxysmal hemicrania (CPH). *Upsala J Med Sci* 1980; 31(suppl):27-33.

43. Campbell JK: The current status of histamine desensitization in the treatment of cluster headache: proceedings of the course on cluster headache, read at the American Association for the Study of Headache, New Orleans, LA, June 1982.

44. Ekbom KA: Heart rate, blood pressure and electrocardiographic changes during provoked attacks of cluster headache. *Acta Neurol Scand* 1970; 46:215-224.

12
The Current Status of Histamine Desensitization in the Treatment of Cluster Headache

J. KEITH CAMPBELL

SYNOPSIS

Histamine desensitization is not an effective treatment for cluster headache despite the findings of increased levels of histamine in the blood and urine of patients suffering from this condition. Recent in vitro observations on H_1 and H_2 histamine receptors support the concept of desensitization by "down-regulation" and other receptor changes. Blockade of histamine receptors by two classes of antihistamine drugs fails to prevent cluster headaches. These observations suggest that histamine plays only a secondary role in this condition.

BACKGROUND

When, in 1937, Bayrd T. Horton administered histamine to a woman with a history of severe paroxysmal headaches, he not only devised a provocative test for histaminic cephalgia but began an interest in histamine and its relationship to headache which continues to this day. Whether histamine is directly involved in the production of the pain, whether it is released by other pain-producing mechanisms, or whether it has any role remains uncertain.

Horton, as a result of being able to precipitate a unilateral headache in many patients who would now be diagnosed as having

111

Horton's headache (histaminic cephalgia or cluster headache), developed a technique that he termed *histamine desensitization*.[1-5] For many years, he treated patients with histamine by subcutaneous or intravenous injection and apparently relieved their headaches in many cases; however, his publications are replete with illustrative case histories but contain minimal hard data on rates of recurrence and duration of follow-up. In later publications, he reported that with recurrent clusters desensitization was less effective and more difficult to achieve.[5] Also unclear are the numbers of patients who were in the clustering phase or in the primary or secondary chronic phase of histaminic cephalgia. Personal communications from his colleagues who recall when histamine desensitization was widely used at the Mayo Clinic indicate that Doctor Horton was an enthusiast for histamine treatment, developed remarkable rapport with his patients, and had great compassion for those suffering from this most painful of headaches. The results of such care and the placebo effect are difficult to evaluate, but over the years it became obvious to many of his colleagues that the long-term results of desensitization were poor. The periodicity of histamine cephalgia was not immediately recognized; therefore, spontaneous remissions were likely to have been attributed to treatment. With the studies of other investigators including Ekbom,[6] Kunkle et al,[7] and Rooke et al,[8] the natural history of the condition was elaborated and the chronic phase of the condition was described. The use of histamine desensitization gradually declined and eventually was discontinued, even at the Mayo Clinic where this procedure has not been performed for many years.

Even though histamine desensitization is no longer advocated as a treatment by most "headache specialists," Horton's initial observations prompted an interest in histamine that has persisted into the modern era. This interest has been intensified by the description of techniques for measuring histamine and the development of two classes of antihistamines that are able to block the two types of histamine receptors shown to be present on many cells, including smooth muscle[9] and neural cells.[10]

THE INVOLVEMENT OF HISTAMINE IN THE PATHOPHYSIOLOGY OF CLUSTER HEADACHE

Horton noted that injection of histamine produced a dull headache in most people but that in those who had cluster headaches it often triggered an attack identical to a spontaneous episode. Horton[11] and others[12,13] also reported an increased incidence of duodenal ulceration in patients with cluster headaches, production of gastric acid reaching values found in patients with the Zollinger-Ellison syndrome.[13] In 1964[14] and in 1970,[15] Sjaastad and Sjaastad reported increased excretion of histamine in the urine of patients with vascular headaches. With these observations, the interest in histamine continued, and in 1971 Anthony and Lance[16] reported finding a mean increase in whole blood histamine of 20% in 19 of 22 patients with cluster headaches, whether the attacks were spontaneous or induced by nitroglycerin or alcohol.

With improvement in measuring techniques, the increased levels of blood and urine histamine in patients with cluster headaches continued to be reported.[17,18] Medina et al[19] studied six patients with cluster headaches and showed that blood withdrawn from the external jugular vein ipsilateral to the headache had a lower platelet count than blood withdrawn from the contralateral jugular vein or the antecubital vein ($P<0.0001$), and in all observations except one (five of six), the histamine level in platelet-rich plasma decreased during the headache. Compared with observations made during freedom from pain, the histamine level in platelet-rich plasma increased a mean of 53%, and the platelet count of blood obtained from the arm during the cluster headache attack decreased. From these and other observations, the authors concluded that strong evidence existed for the presence of a generalized disorder of histamine metabolism in cluster headache and that the target vessels of the head ipsilateral to the pain were sequestering platelets and had an avidity for histamine. Morphologic studies on the increased number[20] and abnormal distribution[21] of mast cells in the forehead skin of patients with cluster headaches gave further support to the theory that local release of histamine is involved in this disease.

These observations must be balanced with reports that have failed to show any significant alteration in histamine metabolism in cluster headache[22,23] and the well-documented failure of antihistamines to relieve or prevent attacks.[24-26] Care must be taken in interpreting histamine measurements in view of the known difficulties in measuring minute concentrations of this substance.[27] Precipitation of attacks of cluster headache by such vasodilators as alcohol and nitroglycerin raises questions about the specificity of histamine as the triggering agent; also unexplained is the lack of headache in patients with basophilic leukemia, in whom serum concentrations of histamine may exceed 300 times normal.

Concurrent with these observations in relationship to headache, a great deal has been learned about the metabolism and mode of action of histamine during the last few years. Histamine has been shown to be the chemical mediator of cutaneous pain[28] and to be a much more potent vasodilator when applied to the outside of a vessel than when it is perfused through the vessel.[29] Histamine is released from circulating basophils and mast cells in response to many liberators including dextran, anaphylatoxin, antigen-IgE antibody interaction, and edema produced by administration of histamine.[30] The release of histamine provoked by antigen-IgE interaction is believed to be the initial step in allergic (immediate hypersensitivity) reactions. The release of histamine, and in some species serotonin, may precede the release of kinins and prostaglandins and may be responsible for the initial edema of inflammation. Schayer[31] suggested that histamine is responsible for the opening and closing of small blood vessels in vascular beds. He proposed that histamine is not stored in the walls of blood vessels but is continuously produced and, upon accumulation, relaxes the precapillary sphincters. This relaxation allows washout that reduces the local concentration of the substance and hence permits reclosure of the sphincters. The possible importance of this in relationship to the vasodilatation in vascular headache remains to be clarified. It has been shown in human lung and basophil preparations that histamine, prostaglandin E_2, and β-adrenergic agents, especially isoproterenol and epinephrine, inhibit release of histamine and increase production of cyclic adenosine $5'$-monophosphate in a dose-dependent fashion. This effect on release of histamine persists long after the other effects of epinephrine have ceased. Historically, Horton[5] noted rapid reduction of symptoms after injection of epinephrine in patients with cluster headaches.

A major advance toward understanding the effects of histamine began in 1966 with the proposal of Ash and Schild[32] that two types of histamine receptors exist. The H_1 receptor actions are blocked by conventional antihistamines, of which mepyramine is the prototype. The actions of histamine not blocked by such an agent are believed to be mediated via H_2 receptors, which can be blocked by burimamide, metiamide, and cimetidine. Both types of histamine receptors have been shown to be present in neural tissue[10,33] and in the vascular bed.[9,34] In studies of dogs, Saxena[34] showed that intra-arterial histamine causes dilatation of the carotid bed, that this effect can be partially blocked by mepyramine (H_1 blockade), and that the residual mepyramine-resistant carotid dilatation can be blocked by metiamide or burimamide (H_2 blockade). If these findings are accurate, it is difficult to understand why the vasodilatation associated with cluster headache is unaffected by H_1 or H_2 blockade[24-26] unless histamine is not responsible for the vasodilation of this condition, insufficient doses of the two types of blocking agents have been used, yet a third type of receptor exists, or the antihistamines are ineffective against locally induced histamine.

HISTAMINE DESENSITIZATION

Clinical evidence to support the concept of desensitization was provided by Browne,[35] who worked with Horton. He showed that the flare resulting from sequential, twice-daily *intradermal* injections of histamine diminished after several days of treatment. The axonal reflex returned to normal within a few weeks after treatment was discontinued.

Desensitization is now a well-described pharmacologic phenomenon, which can be defined as the decreased responsiveness of a tissue to an agonist after prolonged exposure to that agonist. Specific desensitization or tachyphylaxis affects one type of receptor, whereas nonspecific desensitization affects several types of receptors. Cantoni and Eastman[36] first demonstrated nonspecific desensitization when they found that preincubation of guinea pig ileum in high concentrations of histamine or acetylcholine abolished the contractile response to previously effective concentrations of either agonist. Barsoum and Gaddum[37] demonstrated specific desensitization by showing that preincubation of fowl rectum and cecum in histamine rendered the tissue insensitive to this substance, whereas its response to acetylcholine and other agonists was only minimally reduced.

Specific desensitization is believed to involve the agonist-receptor complex and to result from changes in the number or properties of the receptors. Desensitization at specific receptor sites has been demonstrated for many types including muscarinic and nicotinic acetylcholine receptors, α- and β-adrenergic receptors, H_1 receptors,[38] and H_2 receptors.[39] In vitro, a distinction can be made between short- and long-term desensitization, but these are only relative terms because they refer to minutes, rather than days or weeks, during which histamine desensitization has been attempted for cluster headache. Taylor and Richelson[38] have demonstrated that H_1-receptor desensitization of the mouse neuroblastoma cell by prolonged exposure to histamine has a half-time of approximately 9 minutes and a half-time for resensitization, in the absence of histamine, of approximately 13 minutes. Such short-term desensitization does not result from "down-regulation" or disappearance of receptors but possibly from inactivation of calcium channels that couple the receptors with guanylate cyclase.[40] Long-term desensitization may result from "down-regulation" or loss of receptor sites.[41]

Thus, both clinical and experimental findings support the concept of histamine desensitization. The failure of this technique to help patients with cluster headaches appreciably may be due to many factors, about which one can only speculate at present. Such factors may include the rapidity of resensitization of receptors, shown to occur in minutes in vitro;[38] the rapid breakdown of injected histamine once it has been absorbed into the circulation; and finally, the probability that histamine, although involved in the vasodilatation associated with cluster headache, is not the initial or key element in the phenomenon.

Possibilities for research include determining how substances other than histamine, such as nitroglycerin and alcohol, trigger attacks of cluster headache and whether continuous administration of histamine by infusion pump could result in long-term "down-regulation" of histamine receptors.

Currently, the status of histamine desensitization is that it has been relegated, along with many other methods of treatment, to the realm of ineffectual remedies, but continuing research on histamine has so far failed to exclude this powerful agent as being involved in some way in the pathogenesis of Horton's headache.

REFERENCES

1. Horton BT, MacLean AR, Craig WMcK: A new syndrome of vascular headache: Results of treatment with histamine; preliminary report. *Proc Staff Meet Mayo Clin* 1939;14:257-260.
2. Horton BT: The use of histamine in the treatment of specific types of headaches. *JAMA* 1941; 116:377-383.
3. Horton BT: Histaminic cephalgia. *J Lancet* 1952; 72:92-98.
4. Horton BT: Histaminic cephalgia: differential diagnosis and treatment. *Proc Staff Meet Mayo Clin* 1956; 31:325-333.
5. Horton BT: Histaminic cephalgia (Horton's headache or syndrome). *Maryland Med J* 1961; 10:178-203.
6. Ekbom KA: Ergotamine tartrate orally in Horton's "histaminic cephalgia" (also called Harris's "ciliary neuralgia"): A new method of treatment. *Acta Psychiatr Neurol* 1947; 46(suppl): 105-113.
7. Kunkle EC, Pfeiffer JB Jr, Wilhoit WM, et al: Recurrent brief headache in "cluster" pattern. *Trans Am Neurol Assoc* 1952; 77:240-243.
8. Rooke ED, Rushton JG, Peters GA: Vasodilating headache: a suggested classification and results of prophylactic treatment with UML 491 (methysergide). *Proc Staff Meet Mayo Clin* 1962; 37:433-443.
9. Owen DAA: Histamine receptors in the cardiovascular system. *Gen Pharmacol* 1977; 8:141-156.

10. Schwartz J-C: Minireview: histamine receptors in brain. *Life Sci* 1979; 25:895-911.
11. Horton BT: Histaminic cephalgia resulting in production of acute duodenal ulcer. *JAMA* 1943; 122:59.
12. Ekbom K: Patterns of cluster headache with a note on the relations to angina pectoris and peptic ulcer. *Acta Neurol Scand* 1970; 46:225-237.
13. Graham JR, Rogado AZ, Rahman M, et al: Some physical, physiological and psychological characteristics of patients with cluster headache, in Cochrane AL (ed): *Background to Migraine*. London, William Heinemann Medical Books, 1970, pp. 38-51.
14. Sjaastad O, Sjaastad OV: Histaminutskillelse i urin hos pasienter med hodepine. *Nord Med* 1964; 71:526-527.
15. Sjaastad O, Sjaastad OV: The histaminuria in vascular headache. *Acta Neurol Scand* 1970; 46:331-342.
16. Anthony M, Lance JW: Histamine and serotonin in cluster headache. *Arch Neurol* 1971; 25:225-231.
17. Sjaastad O, Sjaastad OV: Urinary histamine excretion in migraine and cluster headache: Further observations. *J Neurol* 1977; 216:91-104.
18. Anthony M, Lance JW, Lord GDA: Migrainous neuralgia-blood histamine levels and clinical response to H_1- and H_2-receptor blockade, in Greene R (ed): *Current Concepts in Migraine Research*. New York, Raven Press, 1978, pp. 149-151.
19. Medina JL, Diamond S, Fareed J: The nature of cluster headache. *Headache* 1979; 19:309-322.
20. Prusiński A, Liberski PO: Is the cluster headache local mastocytic diaethesis? *Headache* 1979; 19:102.
21. Appenzeller O, Becker WJ, Ragaz A: Cluster headache: ultrastructural aspects and pathogenetic mechanisms. *Arch Neurol* 1981; 38:302-306.
22. Sjaastad O, Sjaastad OV: Histamine metabolism in cluster headache and migraine: catabolism of ^{14}C histamine. *J Neurol* 1977; 216:105-117.
23. Beall GN, VanArsdel PP Jr: Histamine metabolism in human disease. *J Clin Invest* 1960; 39:676-683.
24. Anthony M, Lord GDA, Lance JW: Controlled trials of cimetidine in migraine and cluster headache. *Headache* 1978; 18:261-264.
25. Cuypers J, Altenkirch H, Bunge S: Therapy of cluster headache with histamine H_1 and H_2 receptor antagonists. *Eur Neurol* 1979; 18:345-347.
26. Russell D: Cluster headache: trial of a combined histamine H1 and H2 antagonist treatment. *J Neurol Neurosurg Psychiatry* 1979; 42:668-669.
27. Gleich GJ, Hull WM: Measurement of histamine: a quality control study. *J Allergy Clin Immunol* 1980; 66:295-298.
28. Rosenthal SR: Histamine as the chemical mediator for cutaneous pain. *J Invest Dermatol* 1977; 69:98-105.
29. Galeno TM, Knuepfer MM, Brody MJ: Vasodilator response to histamine: dependence upon the site of administration. *Eur J Pharmacol* 1979; 56:257-260.
30. Beaven MA: Histamine. *N Engl J Med* 1976; 294:30-36.
31. Schayer RW: Histamine and circulatory homeostasis. *Fed Proc* 1965; 24:1295-1297.
32. Ash ASF, Schild HO: Receptors mediating some actions of histamine. *Br J Pharmacol* 1966; 27:427-439.

33. Hill SJ, Emson PC, Young JM: The binding of [^{3}H]mepyramine to histamine H_1 receptors in guinea-pig brain. *J Neurochem* 1978; 31:997-1004.

34. Saxena PR: The significance of histamine H_1 and H_2 receptors on the carotid vascular bed in the dog. *Neurology* 1975; 25:681-687.

35. Browne HC: Skin Reactions as an Index to Desensitization to Histamine. Thesis, Mayo Graduate School of Medicine (University of Minnesota), Rochester, 1940.

36. Cantoni GL, Eastman G: On the response of the intestine to smooth muscle stimulants. *J Pharmacol Exp Ther* 1946; 87:392-399.

37. Barsoum GS, Gaddum JH: The pharmacological estimation of adenosine and histamine in blood. *J Physiol (Lond)* 1935; 85:1-14.

38. Taylor JE, Richelson E: Desensitization of histamine H_1 receptor-mediated cyclic GMP formation in mouse neuroblastoma cells. *Mol Pharmacol* 1979; 15:462-471.

39. Adachi K, Iizuka H, Halprin KM, et al: Specific refractoriness of adenylate cyclase in skin to epinephrine, prostaglandin E, histamine and AMP. *Biochim Biophys Acta* 1977; 497:428-436.

40. El-Fakahany E, Richelson E: Involvement of calcium channels in short-term desensitization of muscarinic receptor-mediated cyclic GMP formation in mouse neuroblastoma cells. *Proc Natl Acad Sci USA*, 1980; 77: 6897-6901.

41. Richelson E, El-Fakahany E: The molecular basis of neurotransmission at the muscarinic receptor. *Biochem Pharmacol* 1981; 30:2887-2891.

13
Surgical Therapy of Cluster Headache

DONALD J. DALESSIO

Though the treatment for cluster headache is almost invariably medical, it is not ineluctably so. The headache is almost always unilateral in this disease, often precisely localized in the same site for years on end. Since local pain almost always means local disease, it is natural to assume that a dramatic local alteration in pathological anatomy might resolve the matter in a trice, so to speak. Hence, considerations of surgery arise in this condition.

THE ANATOMY OF CLUSTER HEADACHE

Certain primary observations regarding cluster headache can be set down as constants. Vasodilation occurs, and involves the activities of the autonomic nervous system. If one reviews the neurological anatomy of this area, one is drawn irresistably to considerations of the sphenopalatine ganglion. Nor is this emphasis new. As long ago as 1913, Sluder had suggested that the sphenopalatine ganglion was involved in what we now call cluster headache, but what he termed "sphenopalatine ganglion neuralgia."[1]

The sphenopalatine ganglion, the largest of the peripheral ganglia of the parasympathetic system contains afferent and efferent branches and subserves both somatic and visceral sensation, and autonomic functions. It is closely related to the maxillary nerve, the

119

Table 1. Sphenopalatine (Pterygopalatine) Ganglion Constituents

Sensory	Motor (Parasympathetic)	Sympathetic
Sphenopalatine (V)	Nervus intermedius Parasymph. efferent	Carotid plexus Deep petrosal nerve

second division of the trigeminal nerve, a sensory nerve, and the internal maxillary artery, which circles about the interior surface of the ganglion.

Its afferent connections include branches from the fifth and seventh cranial nerves, and from the internal carotid sympathetic plexus, which coalesce to form the vidian nerve, and the sphenopalatine nerve, which runs over the ganglion and exchanges multiple filaments with it. The efferent branches emerge directly from the ganglion and supply the lachrymal and mucous glands of the face as well as its vasomotor functions.

Thus the ganglion is the relay center for the regulation and interplay of the autonomic nervous control of much of the face, and the interactions of facial and nasal sensations on that interplay.

Given these anatomic data, a series of observations on resection of one or another nerves leading to the ganglion were produced subsequently. These are reviewed in some detail.

Table 2. Sphenopalatine (Pterygopalatine) Ganglion Functions

Vidian nerve
  Greater superficial petrosal
  Deep petrosal
  Carotid sympathetic plexus
	Control lacrimal and mucous
	  secretions and vasomotor
	  functions of face

Sphenopalatine nerves (V)
  Somatic sensation of mucous
    membranes
  Do not synapse
	Branches to lacrimal gland,
	  ethmoidal cells, nose, palate

RESECTION OF THE GREATER SUPERFICIAL
PETROSAL NERVE

In 1947, W. James Gardner and colleagues described their experience with resection of the greater superficial petrosal nerve in the treatment of unilateral headache.[2] Included in their patient sample was an admixture of headache syndromes including some with migraine. What Gardner terms petrosal neuralgia can, however, be reasonably recognized as cluster headache. Gardner outlines his operation in thirteen patients, but one notes that in three of these patients there were attacks on both sides, raising the question as to the accuracy of the diagnosis of cluster headache in this subgroup. Nonetheless, in the patients operated 25% had excellent results, and fair to good results were observed in 50%; 25% were failures. This operation is, in effect, a preganglionic neurectomy, and would not be expected to relieve head pain if discharges of vasodilator impulses originated in the system peripheral to the point of surgical interruption. That is, such discharges might, for example, arise in the ganglion itself.

Complications of this procedure included a dry eye on the operated side, and facial paresis, the latter secondary to operative trauma.

SECTION OF THE NERVUS INTERMEDIUS

Subsequently, in 1967, Ernest Sachs reported on section of the nervus intermedius in "facial neuralgia."[1,3] His patients clearly had cluster headache if one reviews them carefully. Sachs made the point that section of the greater superficial petrosal nerve alone would provide only "an incomplete section" of the components of the nervus intermedius, which contains many of the cerebral vasodilator fibers, as well as the parasympathetic secretory motor efferents to the lachrymal gland and the nasal mucosa. Hence, the surgeon has moved closer to the brain stem itself, for the nervus intermedius contains several nerve fiber bundles including efferent and afferent divisions from the superior salivary nucleus and the nucleus of the tractus solitarius which do not course through the sphenopalatine ganglion. Eventually it forms part of the greater petrosal nerve. Sachs reported that all four patients were immediately and presumably permanently relieved of their facial pains. (Incidentally, in one of these cases a large internal auditory artery may have been impinging upon the nervus intermedius.)

Generally Sachs' patients noted a dry eye on the same side. One had deafness postoperatively "due to retraction of the eighth nerve."[3]

A subsequent paper by Sachs on this same operative technique presented five more cases of nervus intermedius section for a total of nine.[1] Six of these patients were relieved by the operation, apparently permanently. One with severe otalgia was also improved. Two patients were failures. Sachs comments that these occurred when "more relaxed criteria" of a clinical nature were considered and the operation performed.

SPHENOPALATINE GANGLIONECTOMY

Shortly thereafter, in 1970, Meyer and his colleagues removed the sphenopalatine ganglion in 13 patients with intractable cluster headache.[4] These patients were well studied and clearly identified as having that syndrome. Of the 13, seven received little relief, four did well, and two were essentially cured. Meyer, et al, therefore recommended that ganglionectomy be reserved only for patients with intractable cluster headaches. Perhaps even more interesting than the operative procedure itself, Meyer et al were able to provoke attacks of cluster headache in all 11 patients by providing alcohol by mouth. These provoked attacks could be aborted, in every case, immediately, by blocking the ganglion with 1 cc of a 2% lidocaine solution. The authors also examined these ganglia histologically after they had been removed. In only one was there a significant change, with fibrosis, neuronal loss and neuronal degeneration. All of the other ganglia were normal.

CRYOSURGERY OF THE FACIAL ARTERIES

Cook has suggested that freezing with a cryoprobe the occipital, superficial temporal, and sphenopalatine arteries at one operation will benefit patients with "vascular headaches."[5] His report is difficult to interpret. He describes primarily treatment results in migraine but some of his patients probably had cluster headache. Tabular data are not provided. In some of his successful cases Cook has probably frozen the sphenopalatine ganglion itself, and in effect performed a temporary ganglionectomy.

COCAINIZATION OF THE SPHENOPALATINE GANGLION

Since Sluter's time, local anesthesia applied to the sphenopalatine ganglion, or even to the area of the ganglion, has been used as a therapeutic test for the diagnosis of paroxysmal cluster headache.

Barre has now reported a systematic trial of cocaine hydrocloride as an abortive agent in chronic cluster headache.[6] All of his patients had chronic cluster headaches and had not responded to standard therapies. His subjects were instructed in the self-application of cocaine solution to the region of the sphenopalatine ganglion and most were able to learn the technique. Barre believes that the risk of codeine addiction is slight when employing a 5% to 10% solution of the drug, during the cluster headache phase only. Barre comments specifically on the rapidity of relief from the cluster headache which sometimes occurred within 15 seconds to 3 minutes after application of the cocaine solution.

Our group has used a similar regimen in ten patients with intermittent cluster headaches. That is, we have asked our physicians in the Head and Neck Surgery Division to cocainize the ganglion repeatedly in those patients who appear to be resistant to ordinary therapies. None, however, have had chronic cluster headache in the usual sense of that term. The cocainization has been done by the physician and we have not used the self application of cocaine solution as suggested by Barre. Our results are equivocal. Attacks of cluster headache can be aborted, but it is not clear that the course of intermittent, though recalcitrant, cluster headaches is altered. Obviously, in most instances, cluster headaches will cease spontaneously no matter what the physician does.

TRIGEMINAL ROOT SECTION

In a paper published in 1970, and almost as an aside, Stowell remarked that in five cases of chronic cluster headache, the first division of the fifth cranial nerve was divided, "with complete permanent relief of pain."[1] No other details of this procedure are given and no follow-up is provided.

Approximately three years ago, in 1980, O'Brien and MacCabe described three cases of chronic cluster headache unresponsive to a wide variety of drugs, in whom a partial trigeminal root section through a posterior fossa approach was done; in an attempt to produce a reduction in sensation in the first and second divisions of the trigeminal nerve, but not the third.[7] These authors have reported that the treatment was successful in each of the three cases. O'Brien notes that the ideal lesion would be complete loss of sensation in the first division including the loss of the corneal reflex. Failure to achieve total denervation in the first division may be the reason for poor results following lesions produced by percutaneous thermocoagulation of the Gasserian Ganglion. O'Brien does not speculate on the mechanisms by which this procedure is successful, but it is clear that afferents from the first and second divisions interplay with the sphenopalatine ganglion, as mentioned above. The disadvantages of the procedure are evident and include loss of sensation in the first and possibly the second divisions of the trigeminal nerve with its consequent dyesthesias, as well as the loss of the corneal reflex.

CONCLUSIONS

Surgical therapy is rarely employed in cluster headache patients, because medical therapy is almost always successful given the self-limited nature of this syndrome. In chronic cluster headache patients, however, medical treatment may not be successful despite using different drugs in high doses and in different combinations. In these situations surgical therapy may at least be contemplated. The best evidence to date suggests that a treatment plan which produces alteration in facial sensation through trigeminal manipulations would be successful. A percutaneous trigeminal rhizotomy would be an appropriate procedure. Partial trigeminal root section could be considered as a procedure of the last resort. Though it has been reported to be effective, it has the disadvantage of producing sensory loss in the area denervated.

REFERENCES

1. Sluder G: Etiology, diagnosis, and prognosis of treatment of sphenopalatine ganglion in neuralgia. *JAMA* 1913; 61:1201-1206.
2. Gardner WJ, Stowall A, Dutlinger R: Resection of the greater superficial petrosal nerve in the treatment of unilateral headache. *J Neurosurg* 1947; 4:105-114.
3. Sachs G: Further observations on surgery of the nervus intermedius. *Headache* 1969; 9:159-161.
4. Meyer JS, Binns PM, Ericsson AD et al: Sphenopalatine ganglionectomy for cluster headache. *Arch Otolaryng* 1970; 92:475-484.
5. Cook N: Cryosurgery of migraine. *Headache* 1973; 12:143-150.

6. Barre F: Cocaine as an abortive agent in cluster headache. *Headache* 1982; 22:69-73.
7. O'Brien MD, MacCabe JJ: Trigeminal nerve section for unremitting migrainous neuralgia, in Rose FC, Zilkha KJ (eds). *Progress in Migraine Research I.* London, Pittman Books Ltd, 1981, pp. 185-187.

14
Cluster Headache:
The Treatment-Resistant Patient

J. KEITH CAMPBELL

SYNOPSIS

Corticosteroids, lithium carbonate, and methysergide maleate, singly or in combination, are often necessary in the treatment of chronic cluster headache. Inhalation of oxygen will provide symptomatic relief in a high proportion of patients and can be used when preexisting medical conditions preclude other methods of treatment.

For carefully selected patients with intractable cluster headaches, trigeminal root section is an option. Three patients who underwent posterior fossa rhizotomy and experienced complete relief are described.

Cluster headache, especially the chronic form, can be extremely refractory to treatment. The numerous episodes of horrendous pain night and day for months or years demoralize the patient and frustrate the physician.

Ergot preparations, methysergide [maleate], corticosteroids, and lithium [carbonate] are commonly used as prophylactic agents in the treatment of cluster headache, but despite their consecutive or concurrent administration, many patients continue to be affected with episodes of severe pain. Even in those patients whose initial response to treatment is good, relapse is not uncommon. Subsequent clusters and the chronic form of this syndrome are particularly difficult to treat. Also limiting in the selection of a medical program are the contraindications to many of the prescribed drugs; for example, hypertension and peripheral or coronary vascular disease preclude maximal use of ergot preparations and methysergide, and the risks of long-term administration include ergotism, hypertension, myocardial ischemia, and retroperitoneal fibroplasia or other fibrotic complications. Diabetes mellitus, peptic ulceration, and many other preexisting conditions may preclude the use of corticosteroids, and the complications of prolonged use greatly limit their usefulness in chronic cluster headache. With the possible exception of administration of oxygen, all of the other medications currently used in cluster headache have limitations or contraindications.

MEDICAL TREATMENT OF THE RESISTANT PATIENT

For those who fail to respond to prophylactic ergots or methysergide, the author usually prescribes prednisone, using an *arbitrary* tapering course of 18 days, starting with 60 mg daily and followed by a 10 mg reduction every fourth day. Side effects from this regimen are minimal; therefore, the course can be repeated several times a year with little risk to the patient. This tapering course can be given at the same time as methysergide with no increased risk. Frequently, the pain recurs as the dosage approaches the lower values. If the patient's past history suggests that the cluster will likely be of limited duration, the course of corticosteroids is resumed at the 60-mg daily level and repeated. After two consecutive or two overlapping courses of corticosteroids, or if the patient is clearly in the chronic stage of cluster headache, use of corticosteroids is discontinued and lithium is substituted, either alone or with methysergide. The details of administration of lithium have been described by Kudrow[1] and Ekbom.[2] Primary or secondary failure of lithium therapy is not uncommon, but occasionally its reintroduction after a few weeks results in improvement. A few patients in the chronic stage will respond to alternate-day prednisone therapy,[3] but in my experience the dose required has often been too high to be considered a safe long-term treatment. An unexplained observation in one patient was an excellent response to repeated short courses of adrenocorticotropic hormone after a poor response to several courses of prednisone.

Combined with any other form of treatment, inhalation of oxygen for symptomatic relief can be dramatically effective in cluster headache. Horton[4] recommended inhalation of oxygen for symptomatic relief, and it was subsequently mentioned by other authors, including Graham,[5] but did not gain wide popularity until 1978 when Janks[6] reported his personal experience with this mode of treatment. Kudrow[7] reported in detail on inhalation of oxygen and showed that with this therapy up to 75% of patients obtained substantial relief. The chronic sufferers older than 49 years of age obtained the least benefit; however, even in this group, 57% were helped.

SURGICAL TREATMENT OF THE RESISTANT PATIENT

In 1980 O'Brien and MacCabe[8] reported that partial section of the trigeminal sensory root for unremitting migrainous neuralgia (cluster headache) in three patients resulted in complete relief of pain with no complications. One of the patients continued to have episodic aching in the ipsilateral cheek, suggesting that the attacks were still occurring but were not perceived as pain. Interruption of the sensory fibers of the fifth cranial nerve by root section or injection of alcohol into the gasserian ganglion has been advocated on previous occasions and seems to have been successful, but this procedure has never been widely performed. Wilfred Harris[9] reported on five patients who had had injection of alcohol into the medial aspect of the gasserian ganglion and resultant relief of pain, but in only two patients was the follow-up long enough to be significant. McArdle[10] stated that Harris subsequently performed the procedure on "very many more and was very pleased with the results." He also referred to an article by Dott[11] in which the author stated he had always noted alleviation of pain after interruption of the trigeminal nerve. McArdle added, however, that he had examined one of Dott's patients approximately eight years postoperatively who still had mild persistent attacks despite complete anesthesia of the affected area. Horton[12] reported that an attack of cluster headache could still be precipitated by the injection of histamine in a patient who had undergone complete section of the fifth cranial nerve, even though the diffuse headache that always follows such administration was felt only contralateral to the surgical site. McArdle[10] indicated his own preference for trigeminal root section or injection of alcohol into the ganglion in chronic migrainous neuralgia and indicated that he had done "about six or seven of these injections over the last five or six years, so far with complete success."

Because of the encouraging results of O'Brien and MacCabe,[8] three men seen at the Mayo Clinic with intractable cluster headache were subjected to trigeminal root section.

REPORT OF MAYO CLINIC CASES

Case One

A 32-year-old male dental technician began to have episodes of severe pain behind the right eye at age 19 years, four days after an automobile accident in which he struck the right side of his head. The pain was described as knifelike and so severe that he would bang his head on the wall. Treatment with ergots and methysergide was ineffective.

In 1969, at age 22 years, he underwent division of the right supraorbital nerve in Canada and experienced brief relief; later in that same year, he had ligation of the superficial temporal artery but noted no amelioration of pain. In 1971 the greater superficial petrosal nerve was divided, and for five years he was completely free from pain. The attacks then recurred and gradually increased in severity and frequency. For the five years before he was examined at the Mayo Clinic, he had two to four attacks per day, except for a period of several months each year when the attacks ceased spontaneously. Treatments with ergots, lithium, methysergide, phenytoin, antidepressants, pizotifen, and cyproheptadine were ineffective. Results of a neurological examination were normal except for an area of incomplete sensory loss over the right side of the forehead.

In October 1980 he underwent a partial (80%) section of the right trigeminal root through a suboccipital craniectomy (Dr. Edward R. Laws, Jr.). Postoperatively, he had decreased sensation throughout the distribution of the fifth cranial nerve but had retention of the corneal reflex. He has been completely free from pain in the 39 months since the surgical procedure. He believes that he still has the attacks, but they are painless. He has begun a new job, is very pleased with the results of the operation, and is not troubled by the facial numbness.

Case Two

A male glazier, age 40 years, had begun having right-sided cluster headaches at the age of 32 years. Initially, they occurred once every 24 hours, but for the 4 years before operation he usually had three attacks daily and occasionally had as many as six episodes in a day. Apart from 2 months of relief during therapy with lithium, he had not had any pain-free periods. Almost all attacks developed during the night. The pain was maximal around the eye but was also felt in the cheek and temple. Consumption of alcohol would precipitate an attack within minutes.

Amitriptyline, methysergide, propranolol, ergotamine tartrate with and without caffeine, indomethacin, phenytoin, carbamazepine, lithium, prednisone, and dihydroergotamine, singly and in various combinations, yielded no benefit. Inhalation of oxygen gave minimal relief.

Before coming to the Mayo Clinic, he had undergone computed tomography of the head and cerebral angiography, both of which revealed normal findings. In April 1981 he underwent a right trigeminal rhizotomy through a posterior fossa approach (Dr. Edward R. Laws, Jr.). Postoperatively, the corneal reflex was absent and there was analgesia of the entire distribution of the fifth cranial nerve, but he could appreciate firm pressure over the entire face.

During the first postoperative year, he had no attacks of pain, but he recently had a painless episode of ptosis and unilateral tearing. He is extremely pleased with the results of the operation but is somewhat troubled by a retro-orbital tingling sensation. He has continued as a glazier and has had no problems with the anesthetic right cornea. Follow-up to February 1984 indicates he is still free from pain.

Case Three

A 39-year-old man had suffered from left-sided cluster headaches since age 32 years. Initially, he had a partial response to methysergide. In 1975 he was examined at the Mayo Clinic and inhalation of oxygen was prescribed. This treatment resulted in abatement of the attacks as long as he also took methysergide, but in 1976 he had a myocardial infarction and was advised to discontinue use of this preparation. Subsequently treatment with lithium, prednisone, and other agents produced no relief. In 1979 his attacks became more severe and more frequent, and oxygen became ineffective for most of them. He was informed of the possibility of a trigeminal root section and in March 1981 underwent this procedure in his hometown.

In February 1984 he reported that he had not had a cluster headache since immediately before the operation one year previously. He does not have episodic ptosis, nasal stuffiness, or corneal injection.

DISCUSSION

Trigeminal root section or injection of alcohol into the gasserian ganglion presumably interrupts many of the pain pathways for those structures innervated by the fifth cranial nerve, including the face,

sinuses, eyes, meninges, and blood vessels but excluding those structures, mostly posteriorly positioned, that are innervated by the upper
cervical nerve roots. Many of the pain afferent fibers from the superficial blood vessels of the face, however, are believed to enter the
brainstem through the nervus intermedius root of the facial nerve.
This factor may explain the persistence of the appreciation of pain
in the subcutaneous tissues after complete trigeminal root section[13]
and the fact that some patients with vascular facial pain have been
relieved by sphenopalatine ganglionectomy or by division of the
petrosal or vidian nerves.[14]

A major objection to trigeminal root section or a ganglion procedure is the risk of corneal anesthesia, leading to neuroparalytic
keratopathy and loss of the eye. Dandy[15] maintained that this
corneal complication does not occur after sensory root section via a
posterior fossa approach, provided care is taken to avoid damage to
the facial nerve. This statement is in accordance with the suggestion
by Verhoeff[16] that postoperative keratitis is due to damage to the
greater superficial petrosal nerve, which leads to decreased formation
of tears. Fortunately, experience in patients with corneal anesthesia
after surgical procedures for trigeminal neuralgia has shown that
neuroparalytic keratopathy is rare, provided the patient is careful
to protect the eye from dust and is taught to inspect the cornea and
conjunctiva daily for evidence of irritation. Herpes simplex may
occur after trigeminal nerve procedures but fortunately is rare, because it can result in severe keratitis if it affects the cornea. A complication of any trigeminal nerve procedure is the development of
anesthesia dolorosa of the face. This painful sensation is unusual, but
exceedingly distressing.

The encouraging results reported here confirm the findings of
O'Brien and MacCabe[8] and suggest that selective trigeminal root section should be considered for intractable cluster headache. A simpler
operation would be percutaneous radiofrequency thermocoagulation
of the gasserian ganglion. This procedure has been planned for a patient currently being seen.

It is strange that destructive procedures on the trigeminal nerve
have frequently been performed for trigeminal neuralgia but have
seldom been used for cluster headache, which is equally painful and
located in the same region. Perhaps the difference in application is
derived from our clear understanding of the *neural* nature of tic
douloureux and the presumed *vascular* nature of cluster headache.
It is also ironic that the commonly performed Jannetta procedure
for trigeminal neuralgia is for a vascular cause of nerve pain, whereas

the procedure described herein for the vascular pain of cluster headache is a trigeminal rhizotomy.

REFERENCES

1. Kudrow L: Lithium prophylaxis for chronic cluster headache. *Headache* 1977; 17:15-18.
2. Ekbom K: Lithium for cluster headache: Review of the literature and preliminary results of long term treatment. *Headache* 1981; 21:132-139.
3. Jammes JJ: The treatment of cluster headache with prednisone. *Dis Nerv Syst* 1975; 36:375-376.
4. Horton BT: Histaminic cephalgia. *J Lancet* 1952; 72:92-98.
5. Graham JR: Cluster headache, in Appenzeller O (ed): *Pathogenesis and Treatment of Headaches.* New York, Spectrum Publications, 1976, pp 93-108.
6. Janks JF: Oxygen for cluster headaches (Letter). *JAMA* 1978; 239:191.
7. Kudrow L: Response of cluster headache attacks to oxygen inhalation. *Headache* 1981; 21:5-9.
8. O'Brien MD, MacCabe JJ: Trigeminal nerve section for unremitting migrainous neuralgia. Third International Symposium. The Migraine Trust. London. September 17 & 18, 1980.
9. Harris W: Ciliary (migrainous) neuralgia and its treatment. *Br Med J* 1936; 1:457-460.
10. McArdle MJ: Variants of migraine, in Smith R (ed): *Background to Migraine.* New York, Springer-Verlag, 1969, pp 1-9.
11. Dott NM: Discussion of facial pain. *Proc R Soc Med* 1951; 44:1034-1037.
12. Horton BT: Histaminic cephalgia (Horton's headache or syndrome). *Maryland Med J* 1961; 10:178-203.
13. Davis LE: The deep sensitivity of the face. *Arch Neurol Psychiatry* 1923; 9:283-305.
14. Wyke B: The neurology of facial pain. *Br J Hosp Med* 1968; 3:46-65.
15. Dandy WE: Trigeminal neuralgia and trigeminal tic douloureux. *Dean Lewis' Practice of Surgery* 1936; 12:177-200.
16. Verhoeff FH: The cause of keratitis after gasserian ganglion operations. *Am J Ophthalmol* 1925; 8:273-275.

Index

Abdominal discomfort, 22. 100
Aberration, physiologic-biochemical, 80
Abortive agent
    cocaine hydrochloride, 123
        self-application, 123
Acetylcholine, 23, 64, 115
    muscarinic, 115
    nicotinic, 115
Acetylcholine-like activity, 64
Aching, episodic, 129
Acrocyranosis, 91
Activity, 81
Acute, 89, 93
Adrenergics, peripherally acting, 60
Adenosine monophosphate (AMP), 103
    cyclic, 114
β-adrenergic agents, 114
    epinephrine, 114
    isoproterenol, 114
Adrenergic receptors
    alpha, 115
    beta, 115
Adrenergic system, central, 171
Adrenoceptors, 60
    asymmetric, 60
Afferent, 119, 120, 121, 124
    pain fibers, 132
Age, 81, 83, 85, 98
Aggressive, 76
Agonist, 115
Agonist-receptor complex, 115
Alcoholic beverages, 6, 35, 41, 57, 75, 85
Alcoholics, chronic, 32
Allergic, 40

Allergies, 18
    head trauma, 41
    incidence, 40
Allergic reactions, 114
Alleviating, factors, 80
Alleviation, 81
Ambivalence, 33
Amine, 64
    biogenic, 91
    metabolism, 22
    vasoactive, 82
Amitriptyline, 107, 131
Amphetamines, 75
Analgesia, 131
Analgesics, 94
    narcotic, 65
Anaphylatoxin, 114
Anastomose, 60
Anatomically, 71
Anatomy
    neurological, 119
    of, 119
    pathological
        alteration, local, 119
Anemia, 80, 106
Anesthesia
    dolorosa, 132
    local, 123
Aneurysm, 8
Angina, 91
    pectoris, 39, 100
    Prinzmetal's, 83
Anginal attacks, 39
Angiograms, 27, 61

[Angiograms]
  cerebral, 58
Angiographic, 53
Angiography, 51, 58, 62
  carotid, 58
  cerebral, 131
Anhidrosis, 52
Anticonvulsant, 102
Antidepressant, 23, 130
  tricyclic, 25, 98
  (see also Lithium)
Antigen-IgE antibody, 114
Antihistamines, 112, 113, 114, 115
  burimamide, 114
  cimetidine, 114
  mepyramine, 114
  metiamide, 114
Antipsychotic drugs, 105
Antiserotonin effect, 99
Anxiety, 76
Appendicitis, acute, 40
Arousals, nocturnal, 70
Arterial system
  external carotid, 116
  internal carotid, 99
Arteries
  facial, cryosurgery, 122
  intracerebral, 27
Arteriolar, 71
Artery
  carotid
    biofurcation, 57
    common, 51, 52
    dilation, 114
    pulsations, 3
  coronary, spasm, 90
  external carotid, 53, 57, 60, 61, 85
    tree, 63
  internal auditory, 121
  internal carotid, 7, 27, 51, 53, 57, 58,
      61, 62
    cutaneous branches, 62
      terminal, 60
    distribution, 27
    trunk, 60
    vasoconstriction, 27
    wall, 7, 50, 51
  internal maxillary, 120
  occipital, 122
  ophthalmic, 27, 58, 61
  sphenopalatine, 122

[Artery]
  supraorbital, 60, 61
    "resistance to outflow", 60
  supratrochlear, 61
  temporal, 3, 81, 84
    superficial, 18, 63, 122, 130
    xylocaine injection, 84
Aspirin, 77
Asthma, 40
Ataxia, 104
Attack, 15, 16, 17, 18, 19, 21, 23, 27, 49,
      50, 51, 58, 60, 61, 62, 63, 64,
      69, 76, 77, 80, 81, 82, 84, 85,
      87, 90, 92, 97, 98, 104, 106,
      112, 122, 123, 129, 130
  acute, 97
  acute episodic, 16
  alcohol-induced, 22, 104, 113, 116, 122,
      131
  atypical, 16
  behavior, 34
  bilateral, 84, 121
  chronic, 21
  cycle, 69
  diurnal, 71, 98
  duration, 17, 77, 97
  duration, "natural self-limiting", 89, 97
  induced, 19, 58
  morning, 23
  multiple, 24
  nitroglycerin induced, 113, 116
  nocturnal, 98, 99, 130
  onset, 23
  paroxysmal, 73
  periodic, 21
  precipitate, 75
  recurrent, 130
  spontaneous, 39, 49, 58, 112, 113
  typical, 16
Atypical, 16, 19, 24, 25
Aura, 17, 24
Autonomic, 49, 58, 71, 86
  cervical control, 71
  disturbances, 50
  dysfunction, 45, 50, 53
    peripheral, 54
  function, 45, 51, 119
  involvement
    central, 50
    parasympathetic, 53
    peripheral, 50

[Autonomic]
  nervous control, 120
  signs, peripheral, 46
Axonal reflex, 115

BC, 98, 105
Basophil preparations, 114
Basophils, 114
Behavior, 83, 85, 90
  aggressive action, 86
  biochemical, 82
  hibernation, 86
  hysterical, 33, 40, 75, 76
  physiological, 82
Behavioral aspects, 73, 80, 85
  aggressive, 75
  alcoholic beverage, 75
  capable, 75
  coffee, 75
  compulsive, 76
  conscientious, 75
  domineering, 75
  fatigue, 76
  hysterical, 75, 76
  intelligent, 75
  obsessional tendencies, 76
  perfectionistic, 75
  persistent, 76
  phobic, 76
  smoke, 75
  tension, 76
  timid, 75
Beta blockers, 98
Bifurcation, 51, 52, 57
Biochemical, 27, 28, 71, 76, 81
  by-products, 82
Blockade
  H_1 (mepyramine), 114
  H_2 (burimamide), 114
Blocker
  H_1, 63
  H_2, 63
Blocking, 122
  agents, 115
  doses, 115
Blood, 80, 113
  count, complete, 105
  cranial, 39
  flow, 59
    cerebral, 62, 71, 93
    cutaneous, 60, 61

[Blood]
  [flow]
    velocity, 60
  loss, occult, 106
  pressure, 19, 39, 49, 50
  superficial, of face, 132
  vessels, 132
    dilated, 74
Blood-brain barrier, 103
Body type, 75
Boutons, 71
Bowel constriction, 80
Bradycardia, 3, 5, 19, 25, 49, 50, 58, 107
  episodic, 39
  (see also Cardiovascular changes)
Bradykinin levels, 32
Brain stem, 121, 132
Branches
  afferent, 119, 120
  efferent, 119, 120
BUN, 101
Burimamide (H_2 blockade), 114

Caffeine, 131
Calcium
  blood, 81
  channel blockers, 82
  channels, 115
Calisthenics, 17
Cancer, 39, 17
Capable, 76
Capillaries, fingernail bed, 81
Carbamazepine, 131
Carcinoid syndrome, 32, 101
Cardiac, 105
  function, 39
  malformation, congenital, 106
    Ebstein's malformation, 106
Cardiovascular
  changes, 19, 46, 49, 53
  manifestations, 19
Cartotid
  bed, dilatation, 114
  anal, 53, 58
  arrowing, 61
  occlusion, 51
  system, 58, 65
    external, 16
    internal, 16
  tree, 58
Catechol depletion, 81

Causation, theory of, 91
Cavernous, 52
Cecum, fowl, 115
Cells
    ethmoidal, 120
    mast, 63, 113, 114
        abnormal distribution, 113
        degranulation, 63
        granulation, 81
        morphologic studies, 113
        nesting, 81
    neural, 112
    neuroblastoma, mouse, 115
    smooth muscle, 112
Cephalgia, histaminic, 5, 76, 111, 112
Cephalalgias, 26
Cerebral blood flow studies, 59
Cerebral circulation, 93
"Cerebral ischemic" phenomena, 59
Cervical, 53
    disc surgery, 40
Cervicothoracic, 53
Characteristics of, 1, 6, 9, 31
Cheek, 10
    ipsilateral, aching, episodic, 129
    pain, 131
Chemical disorder, 75
Chin, 31, 75
Chlorpheniramine, 63
Chlorpromazine, 98, 107
Cholesterol, 37, 41
Cholinergic hyperfunction, 23
Chronic, 10, 15, 21, 22, 24, 31, 36, 37, 41,
                77, 100, 102, 103, 104, 107,
                128
    primary, 10, 11, 16, 19, 21, 22, 112
    secondary, 11, 16, 19, 21, 22, 112
Ciliary, 53
Cimetidine, 63, 114
Circadian, 69, 70
Circulation
    cerebral, 93, 94
    cranial, 94
    external carotid, 27
    intracranial, 57
        venous (antecubital vein), 63,
            64
Circulatory, 62
Classification, 19, 28
Claudication, 50, 91
    intermittent, 39, 91, 100

Clinical
    presentation, 15, 80, 86
    signs, 8
    symptoms, 19
    syndrome, 23
"Cluster accompaniments", 45, 46, 50, 53
Cluster-tic, 19
Cluster variant, 9, 10, 16
    atypical, 16
Cluster-vertigo, 19
Clustering
    general, 83
    phenomena, 86
Cocaine, 57, 94
    abuse, 94, 95
    intranasal, 93, 95
Cocaine hydrochloride, 123
    self-application, 123
Cocainization, 123
Codeine, 94
Coffee, 75
Cold intolerance, 104
"Cold spots", 60, 61
Complexion, ruddy, 31, 74
Compulsive, 76
Conflicts, 74
Confusion, 104, 106
    mild, 22
Conjunctiva
    irritation, 54, 132
    red, 84
Conjunctival, 54
    congestion, 5
    infection, 18
    injection, 1, 6, 9, 23, 25, 45, 46, 47,
        54
    suffusion, 64
Conscientious, 76
Constipation, 104
Contralateral, 27, 59
    cortex, 59
Conversion configuration, 75
Conversion "V" configuration, 34
Cornea
    right, anesthetic, 131
    (see also Eye), 132
Corneal
    anesthesia, 132
    complication, 132
    indentation, 26
    injection, 131

[Corneal]
 reflex, 124, 130, 131
  absense of, 131
Coronary artery disease, 39, 41, 42
Coronary disease, 101
Corticosteroids, 64, 98, 101, 102, 127
 dosage, 102, 128
 prednisone, 93, 99, 101
 prolonged use, complications, 128
 risks, 102
 (see also Steroids), 128
Cortisol, 65, 70
CHP, 25, 26
 (see also Hemicrania paroxysmal,
   chronic)
Craniectomy, suboccipital, 130
Cranium, 82
Creatinine, 103
 levels, 101
Criteria for, clinical, 1, 21
Cryoprobe, 122
Cryosurgery
 arteries, facial, 122
 cryoprobe, 122
CSF, 57, 64, 81
Culture, 80
Cyanosis, 91
Cycles in, 2, 69
 annual, 69
 circadian, 69
 daily, 69, 70
 episodic release, 70
 fall, 69
 infradian, 70
 nycterohemeral, 70
 pathological, 69, 70
 REM/non-REM, 71
 sleep, 69
 sleep/wake, 70
 spring, 69
 statistical, 69
 variation, 71
Cyclic affective disorders, 102
Cyclical, 85
 changes, 70
Cyproheptadine, 130

Data
 biophysical, 27
 evaluation
  hemodynamic, 65

[Data]
 [evaluation]
  humoral, 65
  pathophysiological, 27
Deafness, postoperative, 122
Decarboxylation, 63
Degranulation, 63
Demographic features, 23
Denervated, 124
Denervation, 60
 total, 124
Depressant, 102
Depressed, 25, 103
Depression, 33, 75, 76, 100
Dermatologic, 105
Dextran, 114
Diabetes mellitus, 128
Diabetic, 81
Diarrhea, 22, 85
Diastolic, 39, 50
Diet, 81
Dihydroergotamine (DHE), 91, 131
 abuse, 92
 dose, 91, 92
 pharmocologic effect, 92
 therapeutic role, 92
Dilation, 27, 114
Dilatation, 58, 61
Disease, local, 119
Disorders
 medical, 31
 nonheadache, 31
 other, 40
  allergic, 40
  appendicitis, acute, 40
  asthma, 40
  cervical disc surgery, 40
  hay fever, 40
  head trauma, 40
  herniorrhaphy, 40
  hives, 40
  lumbar disc surgery, 40
  nasal surgery, 40
  tonsillectomy, 40
  vascular, head, 73
Diuresis, 85
Diuretics, 104
 sodium depleting, 103
Diurnal, 71, 98
Dizziness, 106
Dogs, studies in, 114

Dominance, parental, 33
Domineering, 76
Doppler studies, 60, 62
"Down-regulation", 115, 116
Drinking, 32, 35, 42
Drug interactions, 105
Drugs, intravenous, 75
    amphetamines, 75
    lysergic acid, 75
    mescaline, 75
Duodenal, 38
Duration, 1, 2, 83
    patterns of, 86, 89
Dysesthesias, trigeminal, 124

Ear, 3, 10
    hot, 3
    reddish, 3
Echocardiogram, 101
"Ectasia", 58
Edema, 105, 114
    arterial wall, 59
    mural, 62
        segmental, 58
    periorbital, 19
Education, 80
Efferent, 119, 120, 121
    parasympathetic, 120
    parasympathetic secretory motor, 121
Effusion, pericardial, 80
EKG, 58
Emotion, 86
Emotional, 42, 86
    disturbances, 3
    feeling, 73
    status, 81
Encephalins, 64
    levels, 65
    migraine CSF, 64
Enzymes, 70
Epinephrine, 114
Episodic, 10, 11, 19, 22, 23, 31, 33, 36, 37,
        41, 77, 99, 101, 102, 103,
        104, 107, 129
    acute, 15, 16, 19
    chronic, 23
        clinical features, 15, 17
        duration, 10
        sexual predominance, 17
Ergot, 89, 128, 130
    pharmacology, 91

[Ergot]
    preparations, 127, 128
        contraindications, 128
            hypertension, 128
            vascular disease coronary, 128
            coronary, 128
            peripheral, 128
Ergotamine tartrate, 21, 57, 60, 85, 89, 90,
        91, 92, 93, 95, 97, 99, 101,
        104, 107, 131
    complications, 99
    contraindications, 99
    dose, 92, 99
    headache, rebound, 99
    inhalation, 99
    oral administration, 90
    oral route, 99
    parenteral, 99
    pharmacology, 91
    side effects, 90
    sublingual form, 90, 92, 99
    symptomatic therapy, 90
    therapeutic action
        dosage, high, 91
        dosage, low, 91
    toxic effect, 91, 99
    vasoconstrictive action, 91
Ergotism, 128
Eruptions, acne-like, 105
Erythromelalgia, 4, 5
Erythroprosopalgia, 4
Etiological
    agents, 80, 81
    factor, 84
    mechanism, 84
Etiologies, 10, 62, 82, 87
    psychogenic, 10, 73, 74
    vascular, 10
Etiology, 7
Euphoriant, 102
Exacerbations, 3, 6, 22
Exercise, 17, 81
    tolerance, 105
External cerotid system, 16
Extracerebral compartment, 59
Extracranial, 46
Extradural, 58
Extraluminal, 63
Extrapyramidal signs, 104
Extrasystoles, 25
Extremities, twitching, 27

Eye, 1, 2, 3, 7, 9, 10, 18, 61, 62, 130, 132
  bulb, 3
  canthus, outer, 4
  color, 32, 33, 40
    blue, 40, 75
    hazel, 40, 42, 75
  dry, 121, 122
  eyelid, 1, 2, 3, 7
    drooping, 3, 7, 84
  loss of, 130
  pain, behind, 17, 130
  pupil, 2, 3, 7
  symptoms, 48
  watering, 6

Face, 10, 16, 120, 131
  anesthesia dolorosa of, 132
    autonomic nervous control, 120
    vasomotor functions, 120
Facial, 17, 120
  features, 31
  flushing, 18
  numbness, 130
  sensations, 120, 124
Facies
  leonized, 32, 40, 42, 58
  Leontiasis Ossea, 74
  typical, 32
Father-son relationships, 33
Fatigue, 104
Fever, 86
Fibers
  afferent pain, 132
  cerebral vasodilator, 121
  oculosympathic, 7
  parasympathetic, 54
  pericarotid, 53
  sympathetic, 51, 52
Fibroplasia, retroperitoneal, 128
Fibrosis
  cardiac valvular, 101
  pleural, 101
  pulmonary, 101
  retroperitoneal, 101
  tubular, 105
Fibrotic
  changes, 101
  complications, 101, 128
Flow velocity, 60
Flushing, 18
  facial, 45, 48, 49

Forehead, 1, 16, 31, 74
  ipsilateral, 52
  medial, ipsilateral, 49
    right side sensory loss, 130
    skin, 113
Fossa
  middle, 7, 8
  posterior, 123
    approach, 132
    rhizotomy, 127, 131
      efficacy, 127
Fowl
  cecum, 115
  rectum, 115
Frequency, 1, 70
Frontal, 17
  region, 5
"Functional" syndromes, 89

Ganglion, 120
  cervical, middle, 53
  cervical, superior, 53
  cervicothoracic, 53
  ciliary, 53
  gasserian, 124, 129, 131, 132
    alcohol injection, 129, 131,
      efficacy, 129
      medial aspect, 129
  head
    autonomic, 86
    sensory, 86
  of parasympathetic system, 119
  peripheral, 119
  sphenoplatine, Sluder's, 5, 93, 119, 120,
      121, 122, 124
    anesthesia, local, 123
    blocking, 122
    cocainization of, 123
      self-application of, 123
    constituents, 120
    data, tabular, 122
    freezing of, 122
    functions, 120
    ganglionectomy, 122, 132
      temporary, 122
    histologic examination, 122
      fibrosis, 122
      neuronal loss, 122
    neuronal degeneration, 122
      sympathetic
        first, 5

[Ganglion]
    [sphenopalatine, Sluder's]
        [neuronal degeneration]
           [sympathetic]
               thoracic, 5
Gastric
    acid, 38, 101, 113
    irritation, 106
    secretions, 80
Gastrin, 50
Gastrointestinal, 46
    changes, 50
    disease, 69
    tract, 103
Gastroparesis, 90, 94
Genetic trait, 83
GH (growth hormone), 65
Glabella, 31
Glands, mucosal
    lacrimal, 54, 120, 121
    mucous, 120
    nasal, 54
Goals, achieving, 83
Goiter, noenatal, 106
Granulation, 81
Grouping, 86
Growth, 70
Guanethedine, 54
Guanylate cyclase, 116
Guinea pig ileum, 115
Gun ownership, 36, 41

H_1 (mepyramine)
    blockade, 114
    blocker, 63
    receptors, 111, 114, 115
H_2 (burimamide)
    blockade, 114
    blocker, 63
    receptors, 63, 111, 114, 115
Habits, 35, 80
Hair, thinning, 105
Hairline, 4
Hay fever, 40
Head, 9, 10, 16
    trauma, 40
Headache, 6, 9, 77, 85, 93
    acute, 89, 93
    bilateral, 23
    chronic, 124, 127

[Headache]
    [chronic]
        abortive agent, cocaine hydrochlo-
           ride, 123
        primary, 63, 77
    contraction, mixed
        vascular-muscle, 107
    cyclic, 6
    family differences, 86
    frequency, increased, 21
    frontal, 106
    Horton's, 5, 112, 116
        pathogenesis, 116
    induced, 59
    intractable, 122, 127, 129
        cluster, 132
    low-intensity, 23
    morning, 8, 23
    paroxysmal, 57
        diagnosis of, 123
    periodic, classic, 77
    rebound, ergotamine, 99
    severe, 94
    spontaneous, 59
    tension, 25
    throbbing, 8, 24
        (*see also* Pain, throbbing)
    unilateral, 1, 4, 5, 23, 24, 25, 57, 86,
           111, 119, 121
    variants, 19
    vascular, 4, 8, 9, 57, 64, 65, 86, 113,
           114, 122
        background, 24, 25
        extracranial, 57
        intracranial, 57
Headaches
    intermittent, 123
    left-sided, 131
    muscle contraction, 15
    paroxysmal, severe, 111
    psychological origin, 73
    recurrent, 4, 5, 6
    right sided, 130
Head pain, 5, 10, 11
    episodic, 2
    unilateral, 1, 3, 7, 8
Height, increase in, 32, 40, 42
Hematocrit, 36, 41, 75
Hematologic, 105
Hemianoptic, 26, 36

Hemicrania, 2, 5, 25
  angioparalytica, 3
  neuroparalytica, 3
  paroxysmal, chronic, 9, 16, 19, 25,
          77, 106
    corneal indentation pulses, 26
    duration, 25
    indomethacin
        efficacy, 26
        response, 26
    in pregnancy, 26
    occurrence, 25
    precipitation, 26
    pregnancy, during, 26
    sexual predominance, 9, 26
  tear formation, 3
Hemisphere, 59
Hemodynamics, 58, 59, 62
  data evaluation, 65
Hemoglobin, 36, 41
Hemorrhage, subarachnoid, 8
Heredity, 86
Herniorrhaphy, 40
Herpes, 86
  simplex, 132
Histamine, 57, 62, 63, 64, 85, 112
  acetylcholine
  muscarinic, 115
  nicotinic, 115
  action, mode of, 113, 114
  adrenergic
      alpha, 115
      beta, 115
  blood, 113
  C-14 labelled, 62
  desensitization, 62, 98, 107, 111, 112,
          115, 116, 117
    current status, efficacy, 111
    H_1 receptor, 111, 114
    H_2 receptor, 111, 114
    long term, 115
    nonspecific, 115
    short term, 115
    specific, 115
  infusion, continuous, 116
  injected, 116, 129
  injections, intradermal, 115
  intra-arterial, 114
  intracellular, 63
  levels, 27, 28, 63, 111, 113

[Histamine]
  [levels]
      blood, 111
      urine, 111
  liberators, 114
  local release, 113
  locally induced, 115
  measurements, interpretation, 113
  metabolism, 63, 113
  receptor blockade, 64, 111
  receptors, 111, 114, 115, 116
  resensitization, 116
  serum concentrations, 113
  third type, 115
  urine, 63, 113
  whole blood, 113
  whole blood levels, 63
Histaminic, 76
Histidine decarboxylase, 64
History, family, 37, 83
  genetic trait, 83
  incidence, 83
  migraine, high incidence, 83
  occurrence, 83
Hives, 40
  (see also Allergic)
Hormonal, 50
  factors, 65
Hormone
  adrenocorticotropic, 128
  antidiuretic, 105
Hormones, 65, 105
  adrenocorticotropic, 128
  cortisol, 65, 70
  female sex, 65
  GH (growth), 65, 70
  luteinizing, 70
  nocturnal, 70
  patterns, circadian, 70
  (see also Cycles in)
  pituitary, 70
  prolactin, 65, 70
  RSH, 65
  testosterone levels, 65
  thyrotropin, 70
  TSH, 65
Horner's syndrome, 3, 7, 25, 57, 59
  ipsilateral, 73
  skin, warming, 3
Horton's syndrome, 5

Human milk, 106
Humoral, 58, 71, 102
    agents, 102
    data evaluation, 65
    factors, 62
    triggering, 71
Hydroxyamphetamine, 51
    (Paredrine®)
Hyperactivity, parasympathetic, 55, 58
Hypercalcemia, 81
Hyperemia, 59
Hyperhidrosis, 3
    facial, 46, 48
Hyperlipidemia, essential, 37
Hyperparathyroid, 81
Hypersensitivity, 60
Hypertension, 8, 39, 41, 58, 74, 83, 101,
        128
    intracranial, benign, 106
Hyperthyroidism, 81
Hypochondriasis, 33, 41, 76
Hypofunction, sympathetic, 53, 55
Hypoglycemia, 81
Hypothermic
    islands, 27
    spots, 27
Hypothyroidism, 81, 104
Hypotonia, 106
Hysteria, 33, 41, 75, 76

Ileum, guinea pig, 115
Illnesses, 42
Immune balance, 86
Immunity, 86
Incidence of, 31
Indomethacin, 24, 25, 26, 77, 97, 98, 106,
        131
    dose, 25, 106
    side effects, 106
    tolerance, 106
Infarction, myocardial, 39, 131
Infection
    intracranial, 8
    occult, 105
Inflammation, 114
Inflammatory response, 102
Infradian, 70
Infusion pump, 116
Inhalation, 59
Inheritance, 80

Injectable agent, 91
Insomnia, 22, 100
Intelligent, 75
Internal carotid artery system, 16
Intracarotid, 59
Intracranial pressure (CSF), 57
Intraocular
    pressure, 27
    volume, 27
In vitro, 63, 115, 116
Ipsilateral, 18, 25, 27, 46, 51, 59, 63, 73,
        80, 84, 113, 129
Ischemia
    myocardial, 128
    peripheral, 100
Isoproterenol, 114
IVP, 101

Janetta procedure, 132
Jaundice, 106
Jaw, 4
    upper, 4, 17
    lower, 17

K level, 81, 103
Keratitis
    post operative, 132
    severe, 132
Keratophy, neuroparalytic, 132
Kinins, 82, 114

Laboratory abnormalities, 36
Lacrimal, 54, 121
Lacrimation, 1, 23, 27, 45, 46, 47, 54, 55,
        58, 64
    homolateral, 4
    unilateral, 9
Leonized, 32, 40, 42
    (see also Facies and Physical features)
Leontiasis Ossea, 74
    (see also Leonized)
Lesion, neuronal, third, 52
Lethargy, 22, 104
Leukemia, 105
    acute, 105
    basophilic, 113
Leukocytosis, 37, 41
    polymorphonuclear, 105
Liberators, 114
    anaphylatoxin, 114

[Liberators]
    antigen-IgE antibody, 114
    dextran, 114
Lidocaine, 122
Life style, personal, patient's, 86
Lightheadedness, 22
Light, 2, 3
Lights, scintillating, 84
Limbus, 46
Lipid, 37, 42
Lithium carbonate, 22, 23, 24, 37, 85, 98, 99, 102, 103, 104, 105, 106, 107, 127, 128, 130, 131
    antidepressant, 23
    biological effects, 102
    clearance, 103
    dosage, 103, 104
    duration of treatment, 103
    efficacy, 22, 23
    failure of treatment, 128
    history, 102
    human milk
      secretion in, 106
    indications for, 102
    levels, 103
    long term experience, 103
    mechanism of action, 103
    monitoring, 104
    mood stabilizing agent, 102
    plasma concentration, 103
    precautions, 24
    retention, 103
    salt substitute, 102
    serum level, 22, 106
    side effects, 22, 104
    therapeutic response, 23, 104
    tolerance, 22
Lithium salts, 102
Location, 83, 84, 119
Locus caeruleus, 71
Lower form, 16
Lumbar disc surgery, 40
Lumen, 58
    narrowing, 62
Luminal, 63
Lung, human, 114
Luteinizing hormone, 70
Lymphomatous disease, 80
Lysergic acid, 75

Magazines
    gun, 36
    hunting, 36
Management, 89
Mandible, 1
Mandibular, 16
Manic-depressive, 22, 24, 106
    psychosis, 102, 103
Manifestations, physical, 83
Manipulation, physical, 86
Masculine, 85
    mental attitude, 85
    physical appearance, 85
Mastocytes, cutaneous, 63
Maxilla, 1
Maxillary, 16
    region, 38
Medical disorders, 38
Medication
    anti-inflammatory, 9
    efficacy, questionable, 98
      Beta blockers, 98
      chlorpromazine, 98
      histamine desensitization, 98
      phenyl propanolamine, 98
      tricyclic antidepressants, 98
    nonsteroidal, 9
Medications, 98
    abortive, 97, 98
    analgesics, 94
    codeine, 94
    criteria of patient selection
      adverse reactions, 98
      age of patient, 98
      contraindications, 98
      expected length of periods, 98, 99
      frequency of attack, 98
      previous response, 98
      timing of attack, 98
    dihydroergotamine, 91
    ergotamine tartrate, 89
    meperidine, 94
    narcotics, 94, 97
    oral, effectiveness, 94
    pentozacine, 94
    placebo effect, 94
    prophylactic, 22, 98, 104
      regimens, 98
    propoxyphene, 94
    steroids, 85, 93, 101, 102

[Medications]
symptomatic, 98
Medullary region, 71
Melanin, 75
Melena, 106
Membranes
biological, 102
mucous, 120
Meniere's syndrome, 9
Meninges, 132
Menopausal, 3
Menstrual irregularities, 104
Menstruation, 65
Mental status, 81, 86
clouding, 91
Mepyramine, 114
(H$_1$ blockade)
Mescaline, 75
Metabolism, 63
Methysergide, 22, 57, 58, 102
antiserotonin effect, 99
maleate (Sansert®), 98, 99, 100, 101,
102, 107, 127, 128, 130, 131
contraindications, 101
dosage, 100
drug holiday, 101
maintenance therapy, 100
precautions, 101
resistance to treatment, 100
serotonin-like action, 101
side effects, 100
long term, 101
short term, 100
vasoconstrictive effect, 101
Metiamide, 114
Microscopy, light, 63
Migraine, 5, 6, 7, 8, 9, 10, 15, 18, 27, 28,
37, 38, 41, 45, 58, 59, 60, 62,
63, 64, 71, 73, 77, 79, 80, 81,
82, 85, 86, 91, 107, 121, 122
attack, classic, 24, 26, 74, 84, 85, 86
clinical comparisons, 82, 83
cluster, 9, 16, 19, 26, 85
common, 25, 84, 85, 86
cyclic, 23, 24, 102
auras, 24
average, 23
bilateral, 23, 24
criteria, 24
duration, 23

[Migraine]
[cyclic]
frequency, 23
low-intensity, 23
unilateral, 23
criteria, 24
duration, 23
etiology, 7
focal neurological symptoms, 24
frequency, 23
location, 23
scintillating scotomas, 24
differences between cluster, 86
menstrual, 69
nonclassical, 24
prolonged, recurrent, 24
red, 18
relation to, 79–87
gray zones, 83
point of view, suggested, 83
similarities and differences, 83
variants, 6
Migraineur, 17, 18
Miosis, 8, 18, 45, 46, 48, 51, 54
homolateral, 1, 53
MMPI (Minnesota Multiphasic Personality
Inventory), 75, 76
Modified cluster patterns, 8
Monoamines, 91, 103
Monoamine oxidase (MAO), 23, 82
levels, 23
platelet activity, 23
Mood
changes, 10, 24
stabilizing agent, 102
Morphologic studies, 113
Motor, 120
nervus intermedius, 120
parasympathetic efferent, 120
phenomenon, 4
Mouse neuroblastoma cell, 115
Movement, 77
Mucosa, nasal, 94, 95, 121
vasoconstriction, 95
Mucosal, 54
Mucous membrane, nasal, swelling, 5
Multiple jabs, 24, 25
Mural, 58
Muscle
aches, 100

[Muscle]
cramps, 90, 91, 100
dilator pupillae, 53
smooth, 91
levator palpebrae superioris, 53
Mydriasis, 46, 48
Myocardial, 39
Myosis, 8

Narcotics, 65, 94, 97
abuse potential, 94
Nasal, 54
blocking, 58
congestion, 1, 18
discharge, 47, 58
labial folds, 31
obstruction, 10
sensation, 5, 120
stuffiness, 25, 45, 46, 54, 131
ipsilateral, 47
surgery, 40
symptoms, 18, 47, 48
Nationality, 80
Nausea, 8, 18, 85, 90, 91, 100, 106
Neck, 10, 16, 17
Neoplasm, intracranial, 8
Neo-synephrine®, 57
Nephrogenic diabetes insipidus, 105
Neck, 1
Nerve
cranial, 8
fifth, 120, 123, 129, 130, 131
analgesia of, 131
division, first, 123
root section, 129
sensation, decreased, 130
ninth, 120
parasellar, 8
distribution, 84
eighth, 122
retraction, 122
endings, 91
facial, 132
nervus intermedius root of, 132
fiber bundles, 121
afferent division, 121
efferent division, 121
fifth, 7
maxillary, 119
oculasympathetic, 7

[Nerve]
petrosal, 132
deep, 120
greater (superficial), 54, 120, 121, 132
diversion, efficacy, 130
resection, 121
roots, cervical, upper, 132
sensory, spenopalatine, 120
seventh, greater petrosal branch, 6
sphenopalatine, 120
supraorbital, right
division of, efficacy, 130
therapeutic resection, 54
trigeminal, 77, 120, 123
complete, 132
denervation, 124
divisions
first, 123, 124
afferents of, 124
sensation, loss of, 124
second, 123, 124
afferents of, 124
third, 124
dysesthesias, 124
manipulation, 124
resection, 123
efficacy, 123, 124, 129, 130
partial, 123, 124, 129, 130
rhizotomy, 133
percutaneous, 124
right, 131
root section, 123, 124, 127, 131
efficacy, 130
partial, 129, 130
sensory loss, 124
via posterior fossa, 132
vidian, 5, 120, 132
division of, 132
Nervous System
autonomic, 46, 119
central, 71
internal, 71
central, 22, 70, 71, 103, 106
depression, 106
peripheral
abnormalities, 50
dysfunction, 53
involvement, 53

Nervus intermedius, 120, 121, 132
    efficacy of, 122
    root, 132
    section of, 121, 122
Neural, 50, 132
    dysfunction, 57
    tissue, 114
Neuralgia
    ciliary, 2, 3, 5
    facial, 2, 10, 121
        atypical, 5, 10
        trigger zones, 10
    migraine, 129
        chronic, 21, 129
        periodic, 4, 6, 11
    petrosal, 121
        greater superficial, 6
    Sluder's, 93
        sphenopalatine ganglion, 4, 93, 119
    spasmodica, 2
    trigeminal, 132
    vidian, 5
Neural systems, 91
Neurectomy, 54
    petrosal, greater (superficial), 54, 120
    preganglionic, 121
Neuroblastoma cell, mouse, 115
Neurogenic, 57, 58
    factors, 62
Neurological examination, 130
Neuron
    carotid, internal, 53
    oculomotor, 53
    supraorbital, 53
    third, 52, 53, 54
Neuronal
    degeneration, 122
    loss, 122
Neuropathy, peripheral, 91
Neuropeptides, 82
Neuropharmacological, 51
Neurotoxic, 104
Neurotransmitters, 82, 91
Nitroglycerin, 50, 57, 85, 113, 116
Nocturnal, 70, 98
    arousals, 70
Norepinephrine, 54
Nose, 4, 10, 120
    blocked, 84
    plugging, 6
    running, 84

[Nose]
    stuffed, 84
    watering, 6
Nostril, burning, 18
Nucleus
    salivary, 121
    tractus solitarius, 121
Numbness, facial, 130
Nycterohemeral, 70
Nystagmus, 104

Obsessional, 76
Obsessive, 76
Obsessive-compulsive, 34
Occipital, 16
Occiput, 17
Occupation, 34, 35
Oculo-cardiac, 50
Oculomotor, 53
Ophthalmic-supraorbital flow, 51
Opioids, endogenous, 64
Orbit, 17, 21, 95
    (see also Eye)
Orbital, 84
    fissure, 84
    region, 5
Oscillator, hypothalamic, malfunctioning,
        65
    biochemical disturbance, 65
    neurogenic disturbance, 65
Otalgia, 12
Other factors, possible, 83
Oxygen, 85, 92, 93, 95, 97, 127, 128
    effectiveness, 92, 128
    inhalation, 92, 99, 128, 129, 131
        hyperresponsiveness, 93
    therapy, 92

P-wave changes, 19
Pain, 1, 3, 7, 10, 16, 17, 27, 46, 49, 50, 54,
        57, 59, 74, 76, 80, 89, 92, 93,
        94, 111, 129, 130, 131
    arm, 4
    around eye, 130
    bilateral, 17
    boring, 1, 6, 17, 21
    breast, 4
    burning, 1, 4, 5, 17, 21
    cephalic, 7
    character of, 17, 84
    cheek, 10

[Pain]
   chest, 90
   constant, 5
   cutaneous, 114
   duration, 4, 7, 9, 17
   ear, 4, 10
   eye, 1, 2, 6, 7, 10, 16, 17, 18
      about, 4
      behind right, 130
      canthus, outer, 4
   excrutiating, 4, 5, 21
   facial, 1, 4, 5, 10, 11, 16, 17, 121, 132
      vascular, 132
   fingers, 4
   forehead, 4, 16
   frontal, 17
   hand, 4
   head, 1, 4, 5, 6, 16, 17, 84, 121
      distribution, vascular, 84
   intensity, 93
   jaw, lower, 17
   jaw, upper, 4, 17
   knife-like, 4, 130
   local, 119
   location, 93
   lower syndrome, 16
   mandibular area, 16
   mastoid, 4
   maxillary area, 16
   morning, 7, 8, 17, 23
   nature of, 83, 84
   neck, 4, 6, 16
   nerve, vascular cause of, 132
   night, 6, 9, 17
   nose, 10
   occipital area, 16
   occiput, 17
   orbital, 17
   periodical, 2
   periorbital, 46
   pounding, 1
   pressing, 1
   receptors, 59
   recurring, 2, 4, 5, 6, 9, 10, 17, 127, 128
   relapse of, 127
      (*see also* Recurring pain)
   relief of, 123
      (trigeminal resection)
   severe, 4, 17, 127, 130
   sharp, 1, 17, 24
      (*see also* Multiple jabs)

[Pain]
   shifting, 13
   shoulder blade, 4
   stabbing, 1, 17
   steady, 17, 84
   subcutaneous tissues, in, 132
   teeth, 4, 16, 17
   thalamic, 84
   throbbing, 1, 7, 84
      pulsatile, 17
   tic type, 16
   unilateral, 9, 10, 17, 21
   upper syndrome, 16
   variable, 10
   vascular, 3, 133
   walking, 6
Palate, soft, 4, 120
Palsy, sympathetic, 58
Pancreatitis, 106
Papules, hyperkeratotic, 105
Paralysis, oculosympathetic, 48
Parasympathetic, 16, 19, 45, 50, 55, 119, 120
   hyperactivity, 58
   impulses, 6
   involvement, 53
Paresis, facial, 121
Paresthesia
   of extremities, 91
   unilateral, 9
Paresthesias, contralateral, 27
Paroxysmal, 25, 57, 73
Paroxysms, 2
Pathogenesis, 8, 50, 64, 95, 116
Pathogenetic mucosa, 95
Pathognomonic, 27, 28, 81
Pathological, 69, 70, 119
Pathology, 80
   cyclical, 70, 81
   eyes, 10
   lesion, 81
   nose, 10
   pharynx, 10
   sinuses, 10
   teeth, 10
Pathophysiologic aspects, 57
   amelioration, 57
   brevity, 57
   paroxysmal, 57
   precipitation, 57
      vasoactive substances, 57

[Pathophysiologic aspects]
  severity, 57
  unilaterality, 57
Pathophysiological, 27, 28
Pathophysiology, 71, 80, 112
  vascular, 60
Pathway
  distribution, vascular vs. nerve,
    relation to, 83
  neuronal, third, 53
Pathways, trigemino-vagal, 50
Patient, treatment-resistant, 127
  medical treatment of, 128
  surgical treatment of, 129
Patients, selection, criteria of, 98
Pattern
  corneal indentation pulse, 61, 62
  of occurring, 85
Patterns, 70, 83
  duration, 4, 85
  frequency, 4
  (see also Cycles)
Peptic, 38
Percutaneous, 124, 132
Perfectionistic, 76
Periactin, 85
Pericardial effusion, 80
Pericarotid, 45, 53
  region, 45
  (see also Raeder's syndrome)
Periodic, 77
Periorbital, 19, 27
  region, ipsilateral, 59
Permeability, vascular, 71
Personality
  features, 42, 83
  patterns, 73, 74
    ambitious, 74
    compulsive behavior, 74
    conflicts, hostile and aggressive, 74
    efficient, 74
    emotional state, sustained, 74
    insecure, 74
    lack in self-confidence, 74
    overconscientious, 74
    perfection, 74
    position of responsibility, 74
    "type A", 86
Petrous, 52
Pharmacotherapeutic agents
  BC, 98, 105

[Pharmacotherapeutic agents]
  corticosteroids, 98
  ergotamine tartrate, 98
  indomethecin, 98
  lithium carbonate, 98
  methysergide maleate, 98
  of questionable value, 107
  prophylactic use of, 97
  rationale of using, 97
Pharmacotherapy, prophylactic, 97, 98
Pharynx, 10
Phenomena, cyclical, 69
Phenyl propanolamine (Sinutab®), 98
Phenytoin, 130, 131
Phenytoxin, 105
Phobic, 76
Phonophobia, 18
Photophobia, 2, 3, 18
Potopsia, 9
Physical features, 31, 75
  general, 31, 42, 74, 75
  leonized appearance, 32, 40, 42
  masculine (men), 86
  (see also Facies)
Physical manifestations, 84
Physique, 83
Physiological, 51, 71, 73
  reaction, 81
  state
    anger, 82
    arousal, 82
    depression, 82
    fatigue, 82
    hormonal imbalance, 82
    sleep, 82
Physiology, biochemical, 70
Pituitary, 70
Pizotifen, 130
Placebo effect, 94, 112
Plasma, platelet rich (prp), 63, 113
Platelet, 63, 103, 113
  count, 113
  substances, 82
Plexus
  carotid, 8, 20
    external, 53
    internal, 53
  cavernous, 53
  pericarotid arterial sympathetic, 54
  sympathetic, 57
    carotid, 8

[Plexus]
  [sympathetic]
    carotid, internal, 120
    periarterial, 59
    pericarotid, 4, 51
Pressure
  blood, 19
  intracranial (CSF), 57, 64
  intraocular, 27
  of face, 131
Polydipsia, 105
Polyuria, 105
Pontine region, 71
Potassium (K) level, 81, 103
Precipitating factors, 80, 86
  trigger mechanism, 86
Prednisone, 93, 99, 101, 102, 107, 128
  dosage, 101, 102, 128, 131
  safety of treatment, 128
Pregnancy, 65, 83, 85, 106
Preincubation
  cecum, fowl, 115
  ileum, guinea pig, 115
  rectum, fowl, 115
Procedure, Jannetta, 132
Prodromes, 83, 84, 91
  abnormalities, autonomic, 84
    conjunctiva, red, 84
    eyelid, drooping, 84
    nose, blocked, running, 84
    pupil, small, 84
    tearing, ipsilateral, 84
Prodromic, 26
Profiles, psychological, 31, 77, 78
Prolactin, 65, 70, 103
Prophylactic, 97
  agents, 127
    contraindication, 128
  medication regimens, 98
    ergotamine, 99
    methysergide, 99
  therapy, 102
Prophylaxis, 98
Propranolol, 107, 131
  antidote, 104
Prostacyclin, 64
Prostaglandin biosynthesis, 103
Prostaglandins, 64, 114
  E_2, 114
Psoriasis, 105
Psychasthenia, 34

Psychologic factors, 73, 74
Psychological
  aspects, 73, 76, 80
    crisis, 75, 76
    conflict, 74
    dependency, 74, 75
    emotional upset, 74
    inadequacy, 74
    stress, 74, 75, 76
    tension, 74
    worry, 76
  characteristics, 33
  patterns, 73
Psychopathology, 34, 76
Psychosis
  manic-depressive, 102, 103
  severe, 106
Psychotherapeutic setting, 33
Ptosis, 1, 7, 8, 18, 19, 45, 46, 48, 51, 53,
    54, 84, 131
  episodic, 131
  painless, 131
  unilateral, 5, 8
Pulmonary spasmogen release,
  inhibition of, 91
Pulse, 27, 49
  corneal indentation patterns (CIP), 62
  rate, slowing, 19
Pupil, contracted, 7
  miotic, 94
  small, 84
Pupillary, 51, 57

Quandrantic, 26

Race, 80
Raeder's paratrigeminal syndrome, 7, 8, 45
Receptor
  histamine, blockade, 64
  sites, 115, 116
Receptors, H_2, 63
Rectum, fowl, 115
Recurrence, 16, 23, 25, 60, 101, 102, 112
Reflex, 94
  axonal, 115
  circuits, 94
  corneal, 124, 130, 131
    absence of, 131
  oculo-cardiac, 50
Regional cerebral blood flow, (rCBF), 59
Relation to migraine, 79

Releasing factors, 82
Renal, 105
    monitoring, 105
    tubules, 103, 105
Remission, 2, 3, 10, 15, 16, 18, 21, 39, 50,
        75, 77, 112
Resentments, 74
Resistance, 80
Response, 57
    capacity, 80
    stress, 82
Rhinorrhea, 1, 4, 10, 18, 23, 25, 45, 46, 47,
        54, 55, 80
Rhizotomy
    fossa, posterior, 127
        efficacy, 127
    percutaneous
        trigeminal, 124
    trigeminal, 133
    trigeminal, right, 131
        fossa, posterior approach, 131
Rhythm, sinusoidal, 65
Rhythms, physiological, 70
Root section, sensory, 132
RSH, 65

Saliva, 80
Salt substitution, 102
Sansert®, 107
Scale
    depression, 33, 34
    hypochondriasis, 33, 34
    hysteria, 33, 34
Scintillations, visual, 26
Sclerosis, glomerular, irreversible, 105
Scotomata, 9, 26
    hemianoptic, 29
    prodromic, 26
    quandrantic, 26
    scintillating, 24
Secretions
    lacrimal, 120
    mucous, 120
Section, 122
    root, sensory, 132
    posterior fossa approach, 132
    (see also Resection)
Sedative, 102
Sedimentation rate, 37
Segmental, 58

Seizures, 104
Sensation
    burning, 18
    "crawling", 47
    facial, 120
    nasal, 120
    painful, 2, 132
    somatic, 119
    somatic (of mucous membranes), 120
    tingling, retro-orbital, 131
    upper area, 17
    visceral, 119
Sensory loss, 119
Serotonin, 64, 91, 99, 114
    level, 27, 28, 32, 64
    neurotransmission, 103
    platelet, 64
Serotonin-like action, 103
Severity, 83
Sex, 81, 83, 85
Sexual predominance, 73
Shunting, arteriovenous, 61
Sides, ability to shift, 83, 84, 86
Signs, 83
Sinus
    cavernous, 52
    disease, 18
    infection, 18
    node dysfunction, 105
Sinuses, 10, 132
Sinusoidal, 65
Sinutab®, 98
Skin, 3, 31, 32, 75
    coarse, 32
    forehead, 113
    orange peel, 32, 74
    pitted, 32
    periorbital, 27
    reactions, hypersensitivity, 106
Skull, 31, 62, 75
Sleep, 103
    disorders, 105
        REM suppression, 105
        sleep walking, 105
        slow wave sleep, 105
        somnambulism, 105
    rapid eye movement (REM), 23, 71
        frequency, 23
        increased latency, 23
        sleep, 23, 70, 103

[Sleep]
    [rapid eye movement]
        suppression, 105
        walking, 105
Sluder's neuralgia, 93
Slurring, 104
Smoking, 32, 35, 41, 42, 75
Sodium, 103
    depletion, 103
    level, 22
    loading, 103
    pump, 102
    retention, 105
Somatic, 42, 119
Somnambulism (sleep walking), 105
Soreness, 18, 94
Spasm, 90, 91
Sphincters, precapillary, 114
Spinal cord, T_1–T_5, 53
Spinal fluid, 80
Spirochete, 80, 81
Spontaneous episode, 112
Sprays, intranasal, 90
Stenosis, nasal, 9
Steroids, 22, 85, 93, 97, 101, 102
    dose, 93
    prednisone, 93
Stimuli, 80, 81, 85
    activity, mental, 85
    alcohol, 85
    histamine, 85
    hyperactivity, sustained
        cessation, 85
    nitroglycerine, 85
    pace, let-down, 85
    stress, post, 85
Stress, 74, 75, 76, 80, 83, 85
    post-, 86
Suicide ideation, 34, 41, 89
Sunlight, 86
Supraorbital, 53
    region, 51, 52
Suppositories, use of, 90
Surgery, 119
Surgical therapy, 119
    cryosurgery, 122
    nerve resection, 120, 122
        greater superficial petrosal, 121
        trigeminal, 123
    neurectomy, preganglionic, 121

Susceptibility, 80
Sweat glands
    face, 53
    supraorbital area, 53
Sweating, 3, 5, 7, 8, 18, 64, 80
    altered, 49, 57
    bilateral, 49
    decreased, 49
    facial, 18
    increased, 49
    ipsilateral, 49
Swelling, sensation of, 100
Sympathetic, 45, 50, 51, 52, 53, 54, 120
    carotid plexus, 120
    denervation hypersensitivity, 60
    hypofunction, 53, 54
    nerve, petrosal, deep, 120
    palsy, 58
    pathways, 53
        artery
            carotid, external, 50
            carotid, internal, 50
        ganglion
            cervical, middle, 50
            cervical, superior, 50
            cervicothoracic, 50
            ciliary, 50
        muscle
            dilator pupillae, 53
            smooth
                levator palpebrae superioris, 53
        neuron
            carotid, internal, 53
            oculomotor, 53
            supraorbital, 53
        plexus
            carotid, external, 50
            carotid, internal, 50
            cavernous, 50
        spinal cord
            T_1, 53
            T_5, 53
        sweat glands
            face, 53
            supraorbital, 53
    system, peripheral, 71
    terminals, 54
    trunk, sympathetic, cervical, 50
    white ramus communicans, 53
Sympathomimetic agents, 54

Symptoms, 80, 83
  autonomic, 25
    unilateral, 21
  contralateral focal, 27
  contralateral sensory, 27
  motor, 27
  visual, 17
    transient, 26
Synapse, 120
Synaptically, 71
Syndrome
  carcinoid, 3, 101
  chronic cluster, 22
  chronic paroxysmal hemicrania, 25
  cluster headache variant, 24
    indomethacin, response to, 24
    symptoms, 24
  "functional", 89
  paratrigeminal, 7
  vascular headache, 45
Syndromes
  cephalic pain, other, 7
  facial pain, 10
  headache, 121
  Raeder's paratrigeminal, 7
    pathogenesis, 8
    prognosis, 8
    sexual predominance, 7
    treatment, 8
  relation of, 7
Syphilis, 80
System, carotid, 65
Systemic signs, 85
  diarrhea, 85
  diuresis, 85
  nausea, 85
  vomiting, 85
Systole, 61
Systolic, 39, 50

T_3, 105
T_4, 105
"T" score, 35
T-wave flattening, 105
Tachyphylaxis, 115
Tear formation, 3, 5, 18
  (*see also* Horner's syndrome)
Tearing, 27, 47, 54
  ipsilateral, 25, 84
  unilateral, 131

Tears, 3, 47, 80, 132
  drainage, 54
Teeth, 4, 10, 17
  lower, 1
  upper, 1
Temperature, skin, 60
Temple, 1, 16, 17, 21, 131
  pain, 131
Temporal, 25
  maxillary region, 9
Tenderness, 18, 94
Tenseness, 17
Tension
  psychological, 76
  state, 73
Testosterone, 65
Tests
  physiological, 51
  pupillary, 51
Therapeutic, 89
  index, 106
  interventions, 41
  maneuvers, response to, 83, 85
  response, 23, 86
Therapy
  acute, 95
  medical, 16, 124
  other, 93
  prophylactic, 93
  surgical, 119, 124
    nerve resection, 120
Thermocoagulation
  percutaneous, 124
    disadvantages of, 124
  radiofrequency
    percutaneous, 132
Thermographic studies, 61
Thermography, 27, 60
  cutaneous, 62
Throat, sore, 4
Thrombophlebitis, 101
Thyroid, 104
  enlargement, 104
  hypothyroidism, 104
  TSH, 105
  T_3, 105
  T_4, 105
TSH (thyroid stimulating hormone), 105
Thyrotropin, 70
Tic, 19

Tic douloureux, 2, 16, 132
Tightness, 17
Timid, 75
Timing, 98
Tissue
    levels, 81
    structure change, 80
Tomography, of head, 131
Tonometry, dynamic, 61, 127
Tonsillectomy, 40
Toxic reactions, 91
Traits
    personality, 31
    somatic, 31
Trauma, 40
    operative, 121
Treatment, 89, 93, 119
    abortive, 100
    efficacy, 78
    "success", 92
Tremor, 22, 104
Trigeminal, 77
Trigemino-vagal, 50
Trigger mechanisms, 83, 86
Trigger zones, 10
Triggering agent, 113
Triglyceride level, 37, 41
Trunk, sympathetic, cervical, 53
TSH, 65
Turbinates, 10
Twitching, 27

Ulcer disease, 41, 42, 74, 75
    autonomic involvement, 54
    duodenal, 38, 113
    peptic, 38, 50, 54, 58, 69, 101, 106
Ulceration, peptic, 128
Ulcers, cutaneous, 105
Ultrastructural study, 63
Upper form, 16
Urinalysis, 105
Urine, 81, 113
    concentration, 105
    histamine, 63
Uvula, 4

Vagal tone, increased, 19
Variant, 11, 16, 21, 25, 26, 77, 79, 86, 106
    atypical, 77
    syndrome, 24

Vascular, 26, 57, 132
    beds, 114
    changes, 86
    disease, 83
        coronary, 128
        peripheral, 101, 128
    disorders, head, 73
    distribution, 84
    involvement, 86
Vasculature
    cranial, dysfunction, 60
    extracranial, 46
Vasoactive, 28
    substance, 57
    alcohol, 57
    histamine, 57
    nitroglycerine, 5
Vasoconstrictors, 95
Vasoconstriction, 27, 61, 91, 92, 94, 95
    cerebral, 93, 94
    conjunctival, 54
    cranial, 94
    nasal, 54
    serotonin induced, 99
    supraorbital artery, 60
Vasoconstrictive effect, 101
Vasoconstrictor responses
    to serotonin, 91
Vasodilatation, 27, 46, 63, 85, 114, 116,
        119
    conjunctival, 54, 55
    multi-focal
        paroxysmal, recurrent, 77
    nasal, 54, 55
    orbit, around, 95
    painful, 91, 95
    paroxysmal, 4, 9
Vasodilator impulses, 121
Vasodilators, 113, 114
Vasomotor, 120
    functions (of face), 120
Vasoreactivity, 39
Vein
    antecubital, 63, 113
    jugular, 63
        contralateral, 113
        external, 113
Veins, scalp, superficial, 18
Velocity, 60
Venules, increase in, 100

Vertigo, 9, 19, 77
Vessels, 114
    carotid, external, 57
    cerebral, 59
    choroidal, 27
    conjunctival, 46
    extracerebral, 59
    face, 5
    facial, 74
    intracranial, 63
    ocular, 61
    small, 60, 61, 62, 114
    swollen, 84
    target (of head), 113
    temporal, 81
Vision
    aberrations, 18
    blurred, 18, 104
    blurring, ipsilateral, 27

Visual disturbances, ipsilateral, 27
Vomiting, 8, 18, 85, 90, 91, 100, 106

Weakness, 22
    unilateral, 9
Weight, 32, 40, 80
    gain, 100
White blood count, 36, 37, 41
    (*see also* Leukocytosis)
White ramus communications, 53

Xe technique
    inhalation, 59
    intracarotid, 59
    intravenous, 59
Xylocaine, 84

Zollinger-Ellison syndrome, 113
Zygoma, 4